# HOW I BROKE UP
## WITH MY COLON

"Wherever the art of medicine is loved, there is also a love of humanity."

—Hippocrates

Am I right
or am I right?

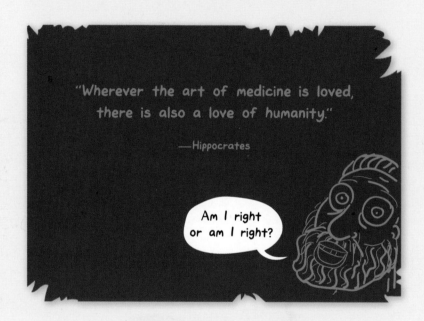

the Awkward Yeti™ Presents

# HOW I BROKE UP WITH MY COLON

## FASCINATING, BIZARRE, AND TRUE HEALTH STORIES

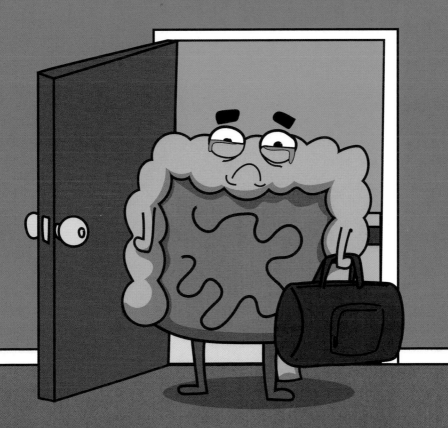

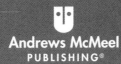

Andrews McMeel
PUBLISHING®

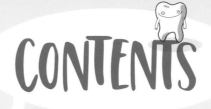

# CONTENTS

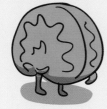

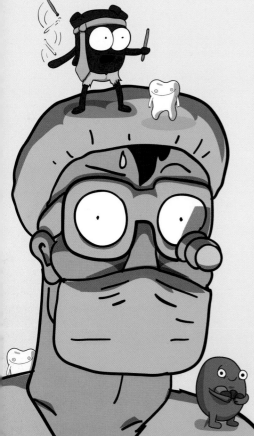

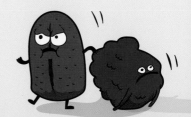

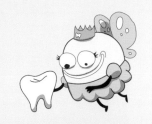

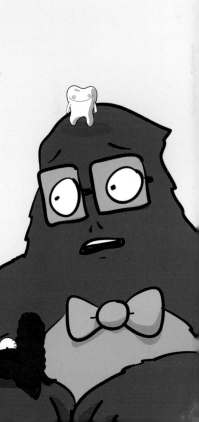

Dedicated to
Calan, Emmett, and Nola

# PROLOGUE

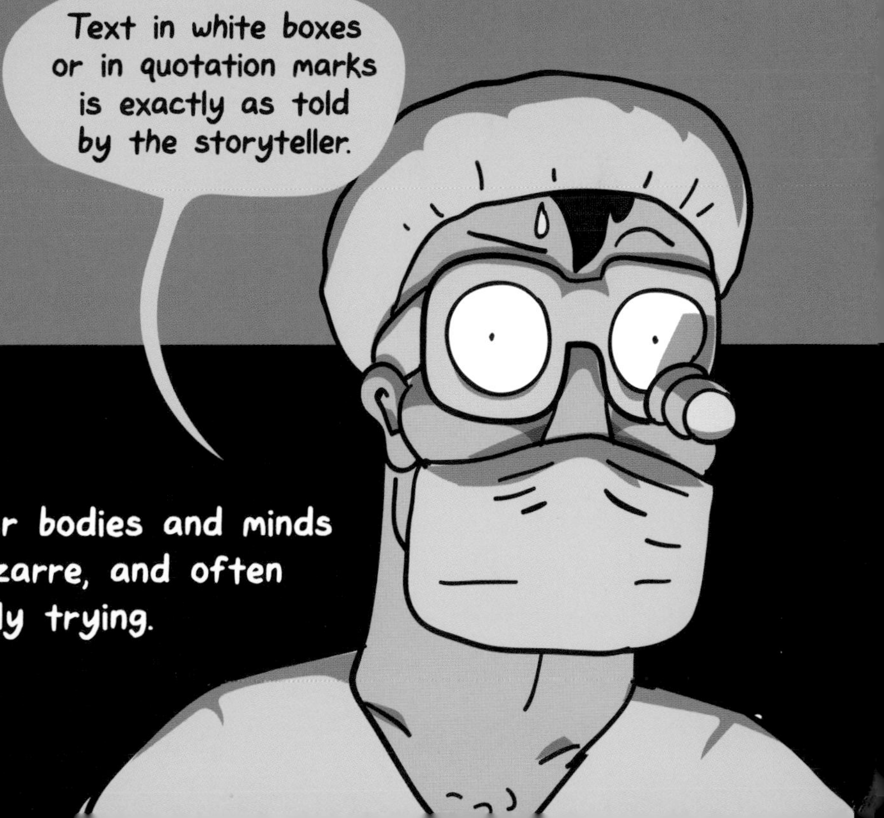
Text in white boxes or in quotation marks is exactly as told by the storyteller.

Experiences with our bodies and minds can be funny, bizarre, and often emotionally trying.

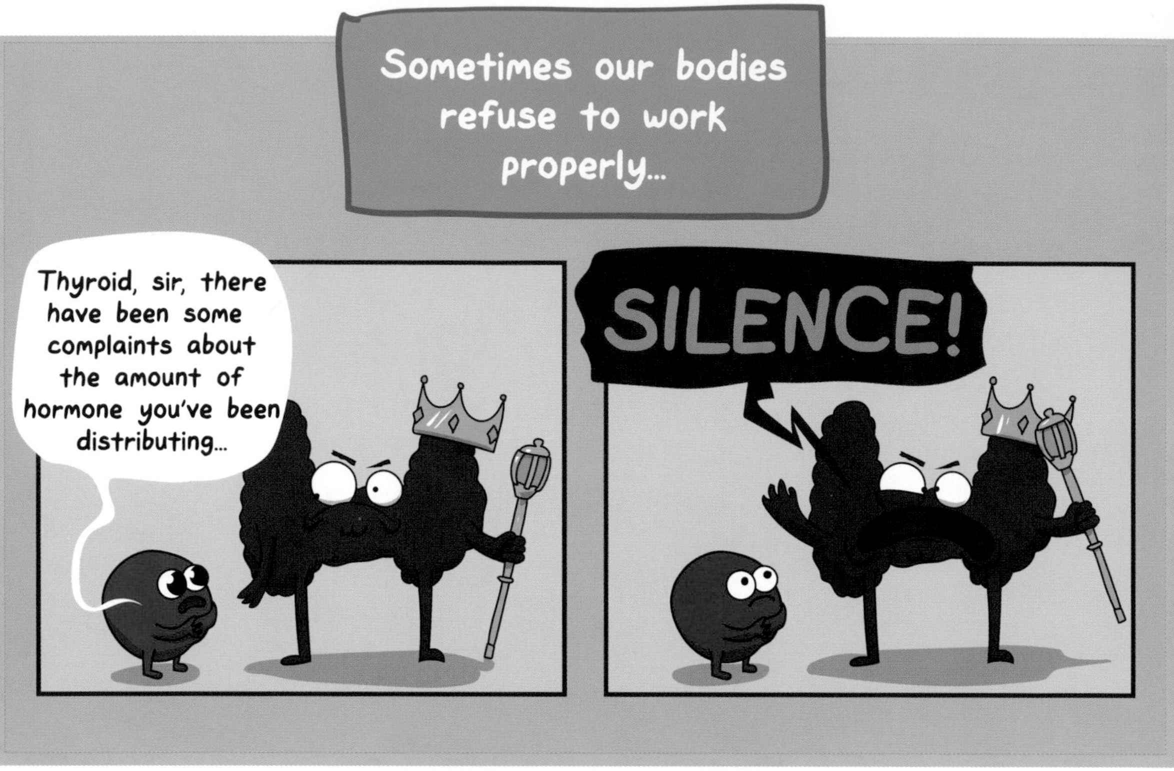
Sometimes our bodies refuse to work properly...
Thyroid, sir, there have been some complaints about the amount of hormone you've been distributing...
SILENCE!

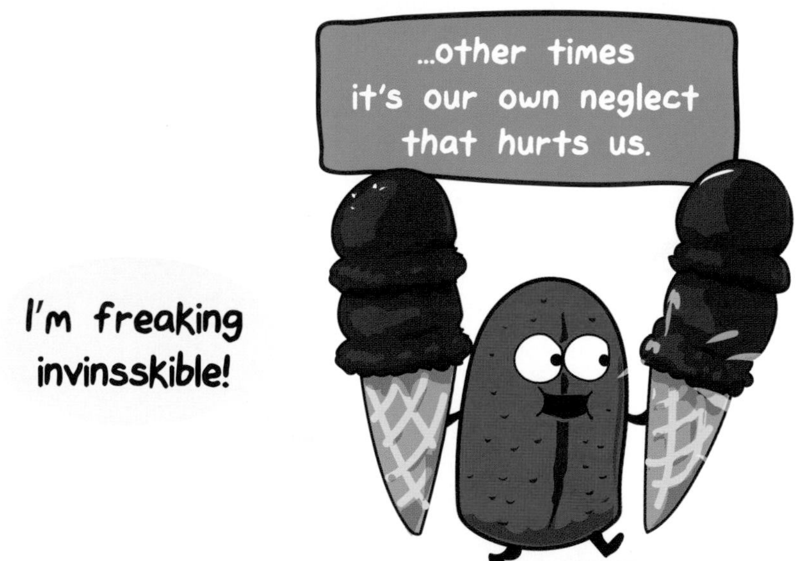
...other times it's our own neglect that hurts us.
I'm freaking invinsskible!

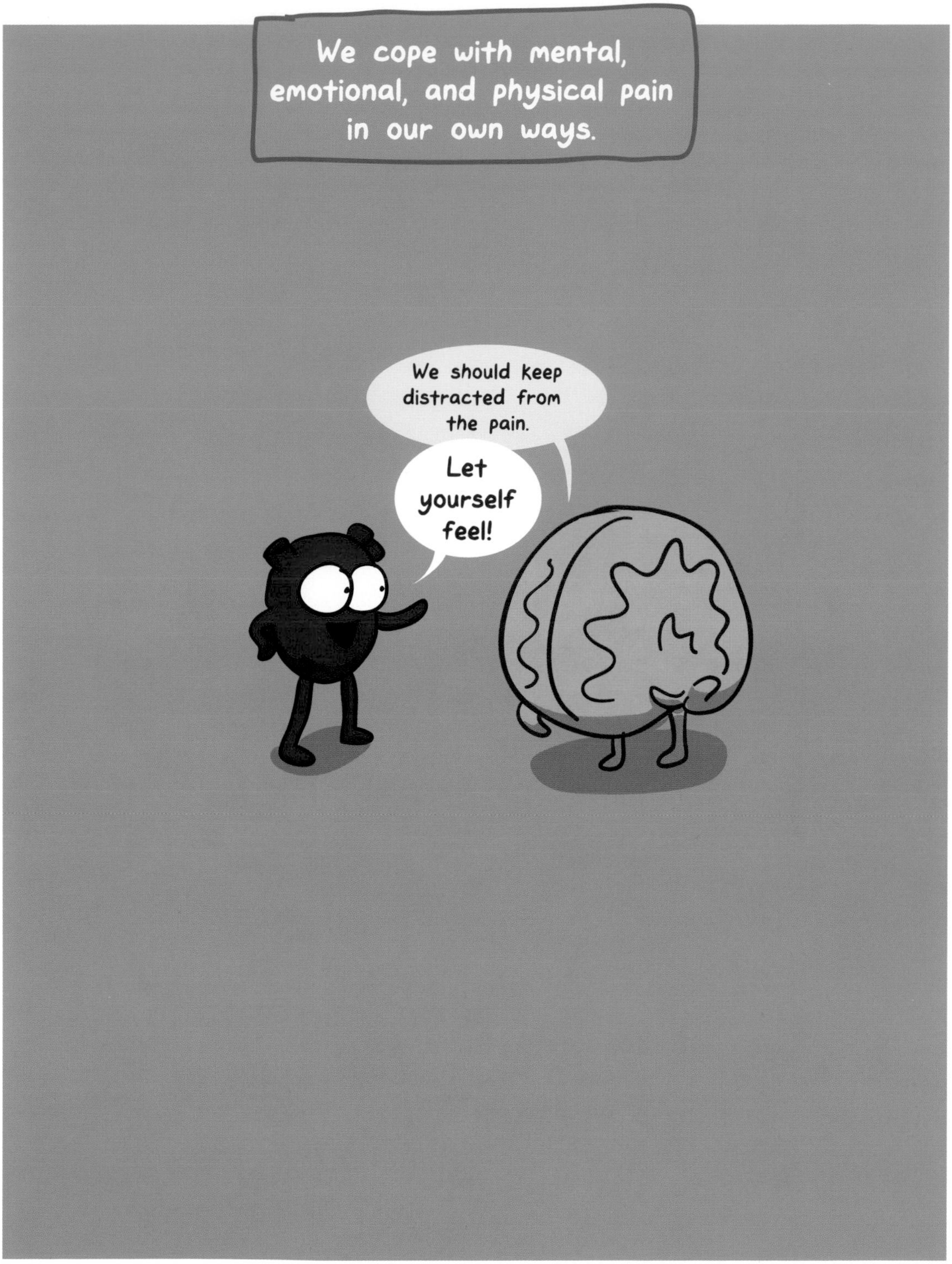
We cope with mental, emotional, and physical pain in our own ways.
We should keep distracted from the pain.
Let yourself feel!

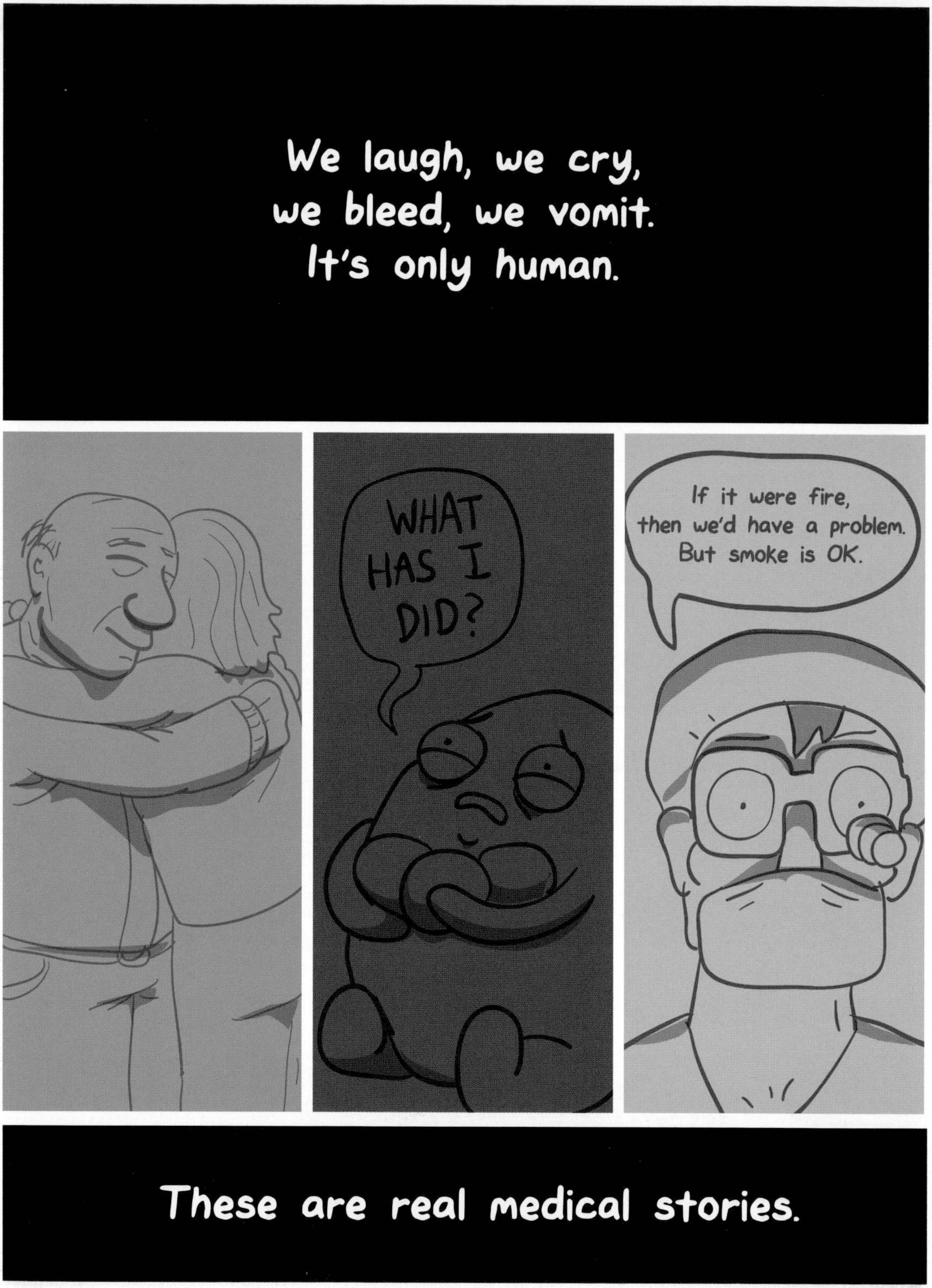
We laugh, we cry,
we bleed, we vomit.
It's only human.
WHAT HAS I DID?
If it were fire, then we'd have a problem. But smoke is OK.
These are real medical stories.

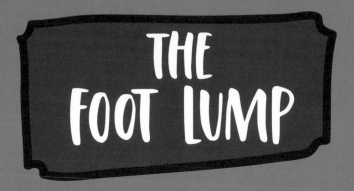

# CHAPTER 1

# THE FOOT LUMP

## told by mattio

I was hanging out on a beach in Rhode Island with a friend, exploring tide pools...

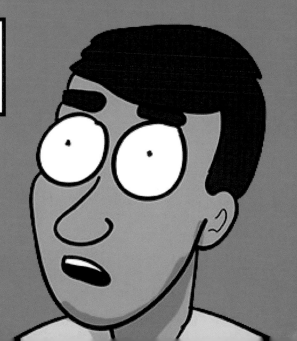

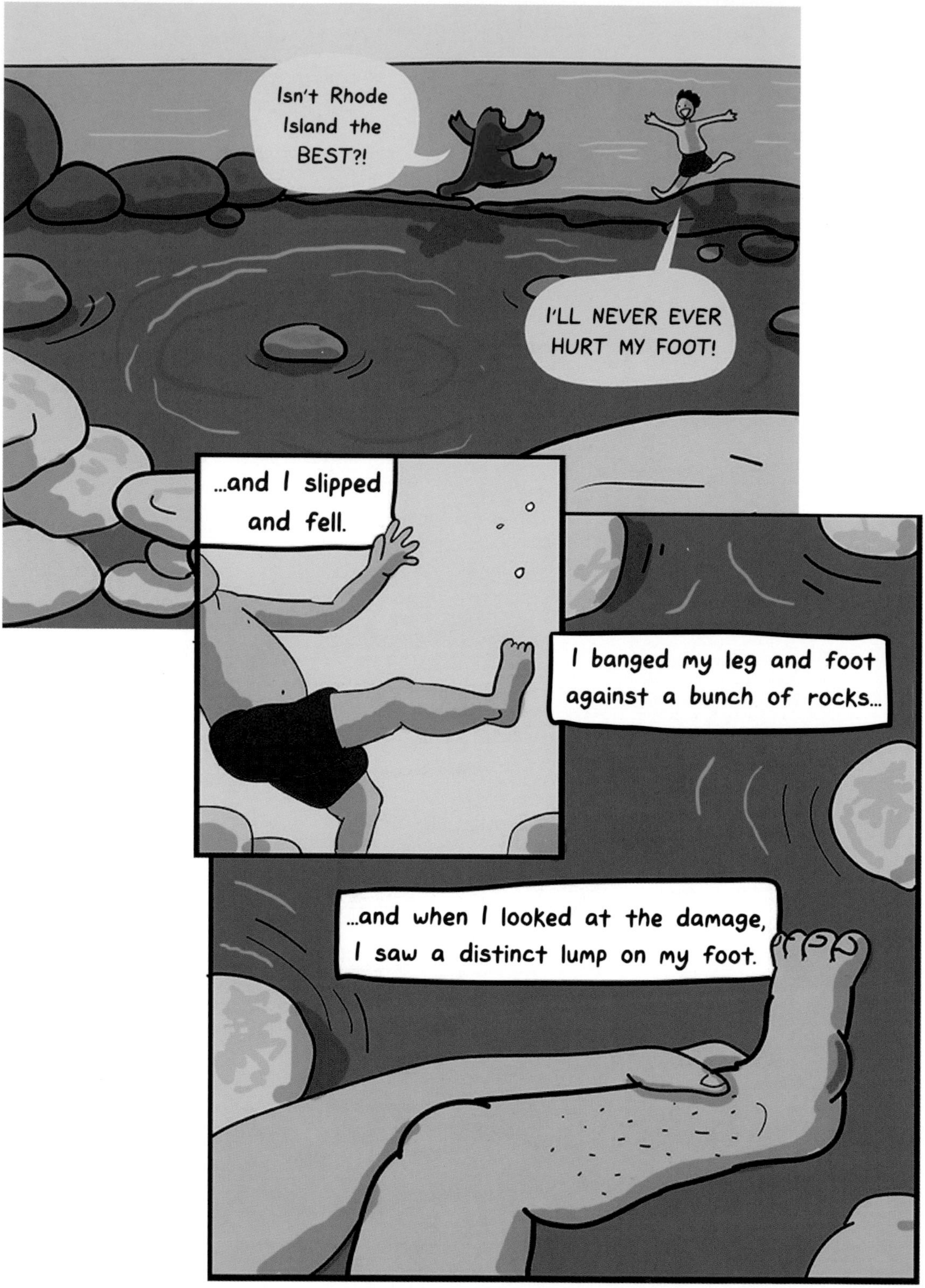
Isn't Rhode Island the BEST?!
I'LL NEVER EVER HURT MY FOOT!
...and I slipped and fell.
I banged my leg and foot against a bunch of rocks...
...and when I looked at the damage, I saw a distinct lump on my foot.

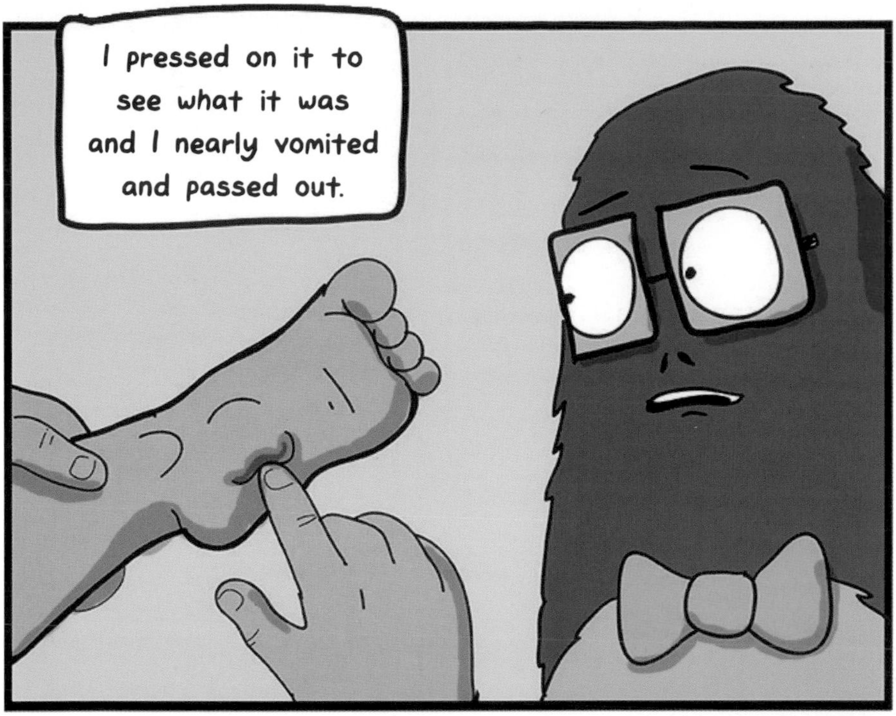
I pressed on it to see what it was and I nearly vomited and passed out.

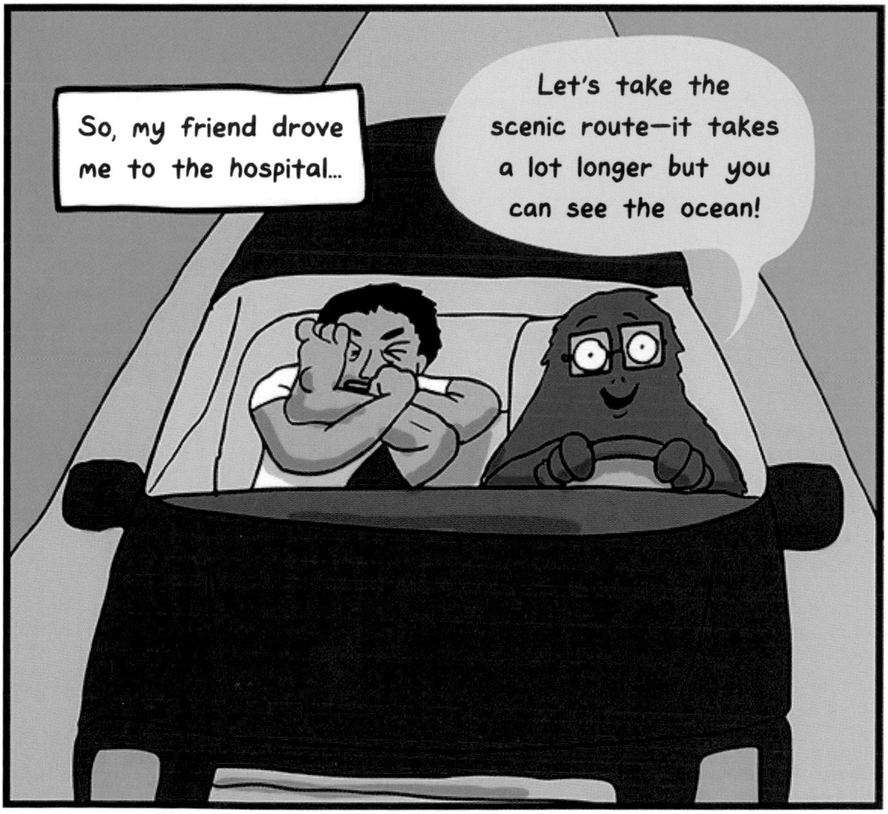
So, my friend drove me to the hospital...
Let's take the scenic route—it takes a lot longer but you can see the ocean!

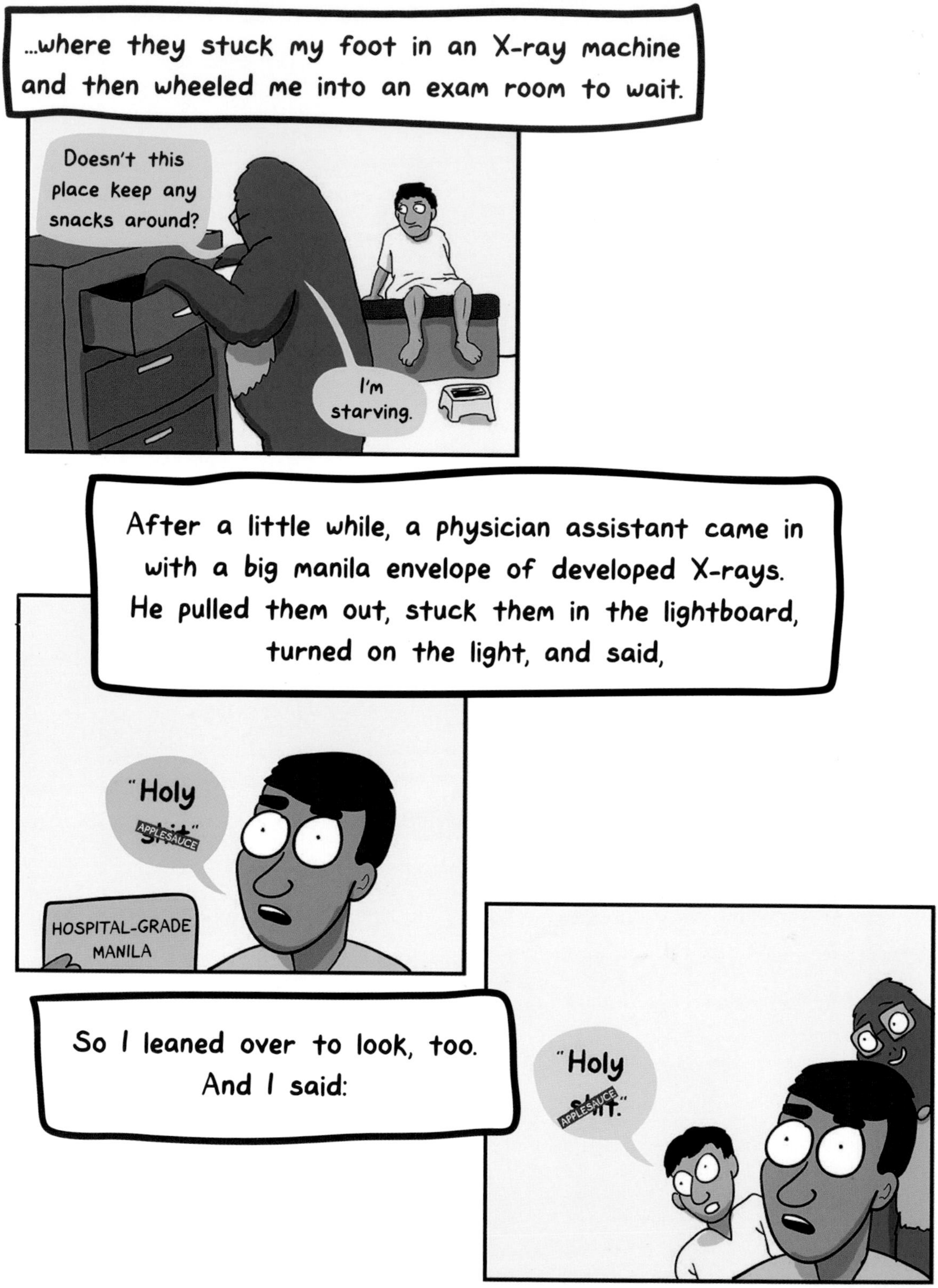
...where they stuck my foot in an X-ray machine and then wheeled me into an exam room to wait.
Doesn't this place keep any snacks around?
I'm starving.
After a little while, a physician assistant came in with a big manila envelope of developed X-rays. He pulled them out, stuck them in the lightboard, turned on the light, and said,
"Holy APPLESAUCE"
HOSPITAL-GRADE MANILA
So I leaned over to look, too. And I said:
"Holy APPLESAUCE."

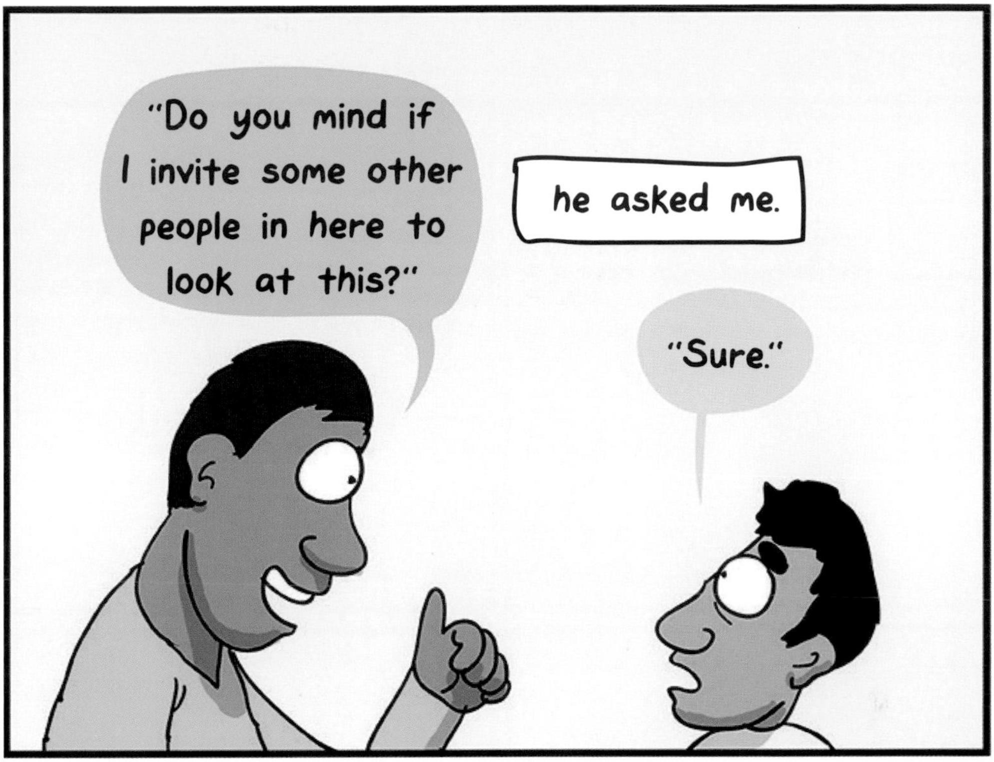
"Do you mind if I invite some other people in here to look at this?"
he asked me.
"Sure."

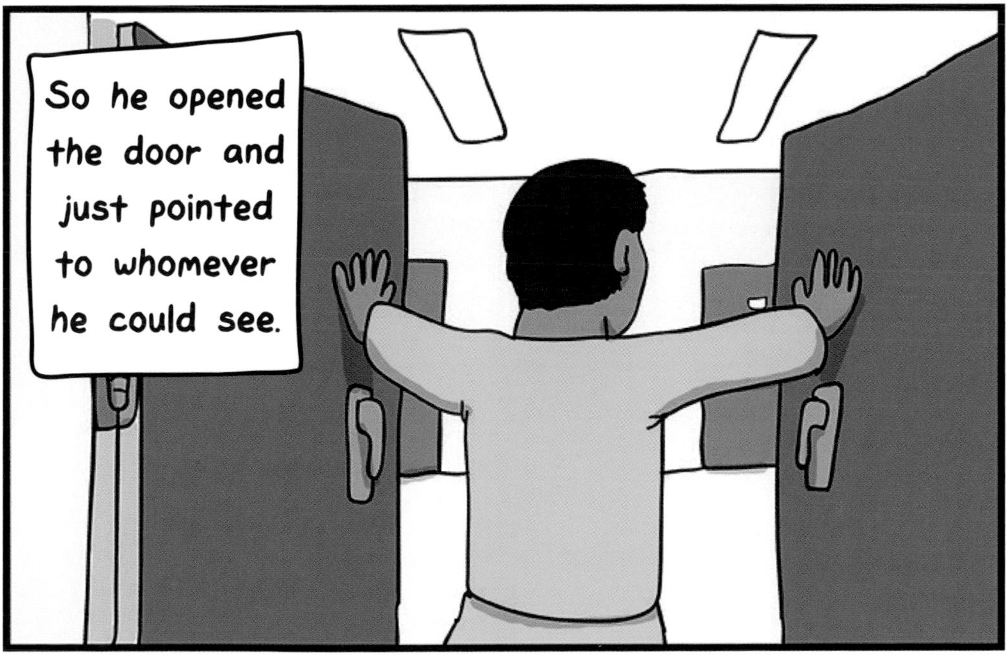
So he opened the door and just pointed to whomever he could see.

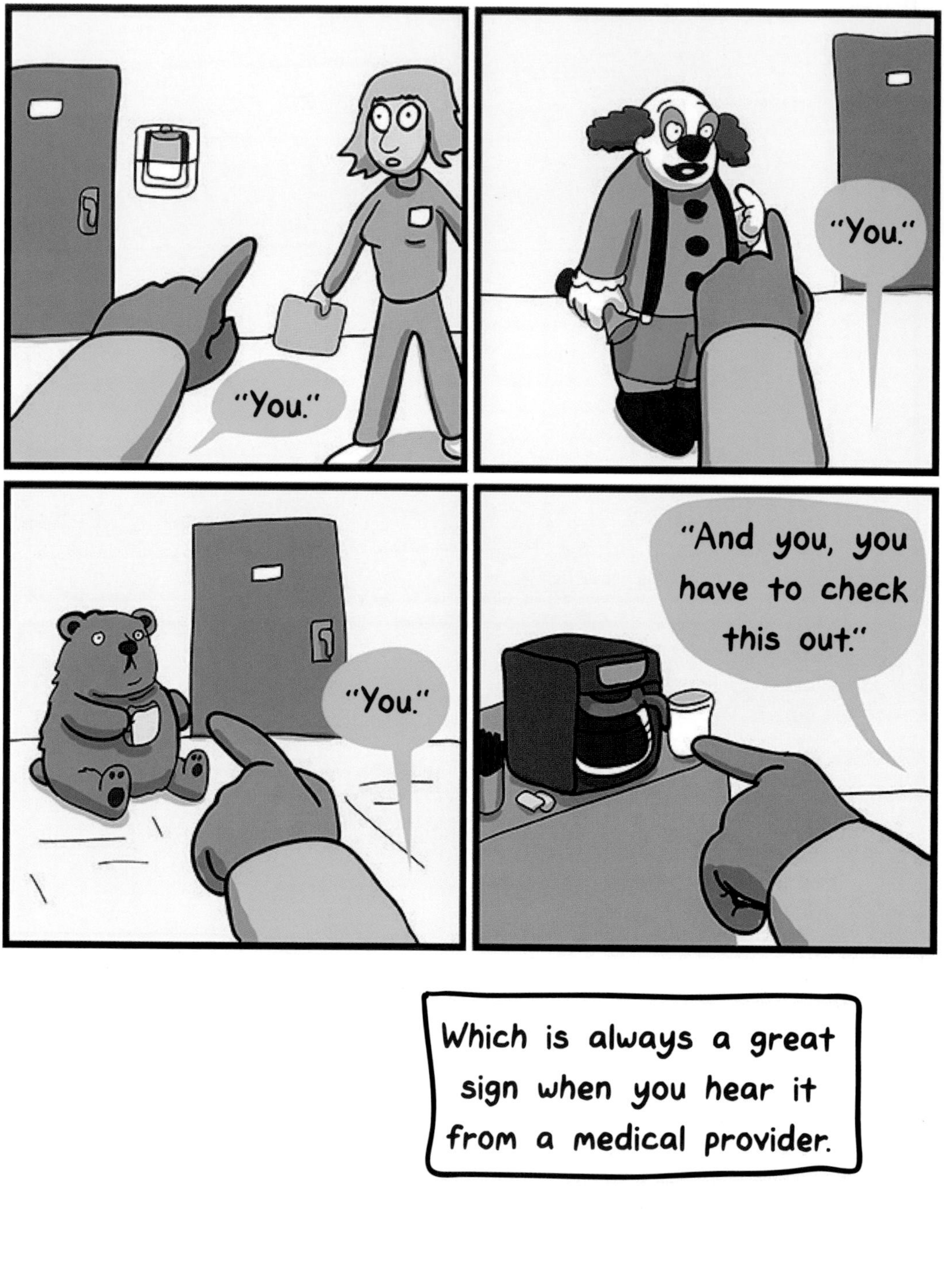
"You."
"You."
"You."
"And you, you have to check this out."
Which is always a great sign when you hear it from a medical provider.

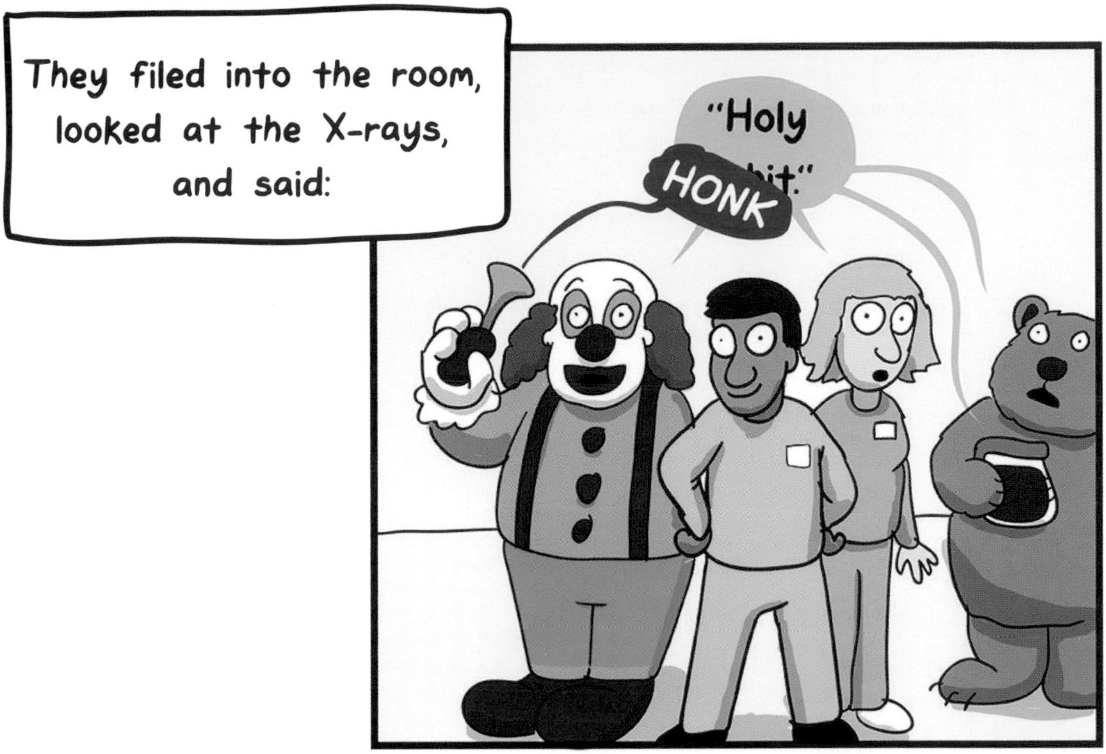
They filed into the room, looked at the X-rays, and said:
HONK
“Holy
hit.”

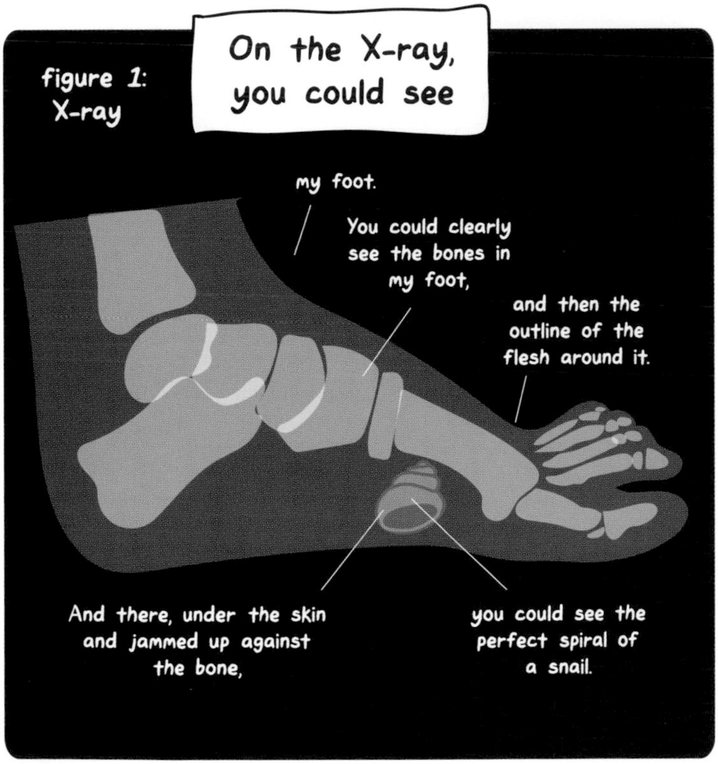
figure 1: X-ray
On the X-ray, you could see
my foot.
You could clearly see the bones in my foot,
and then the outline of the flesh around it.
And there, under the skin and jammed up against the bone,
you could see the perfect spiral of a snail.

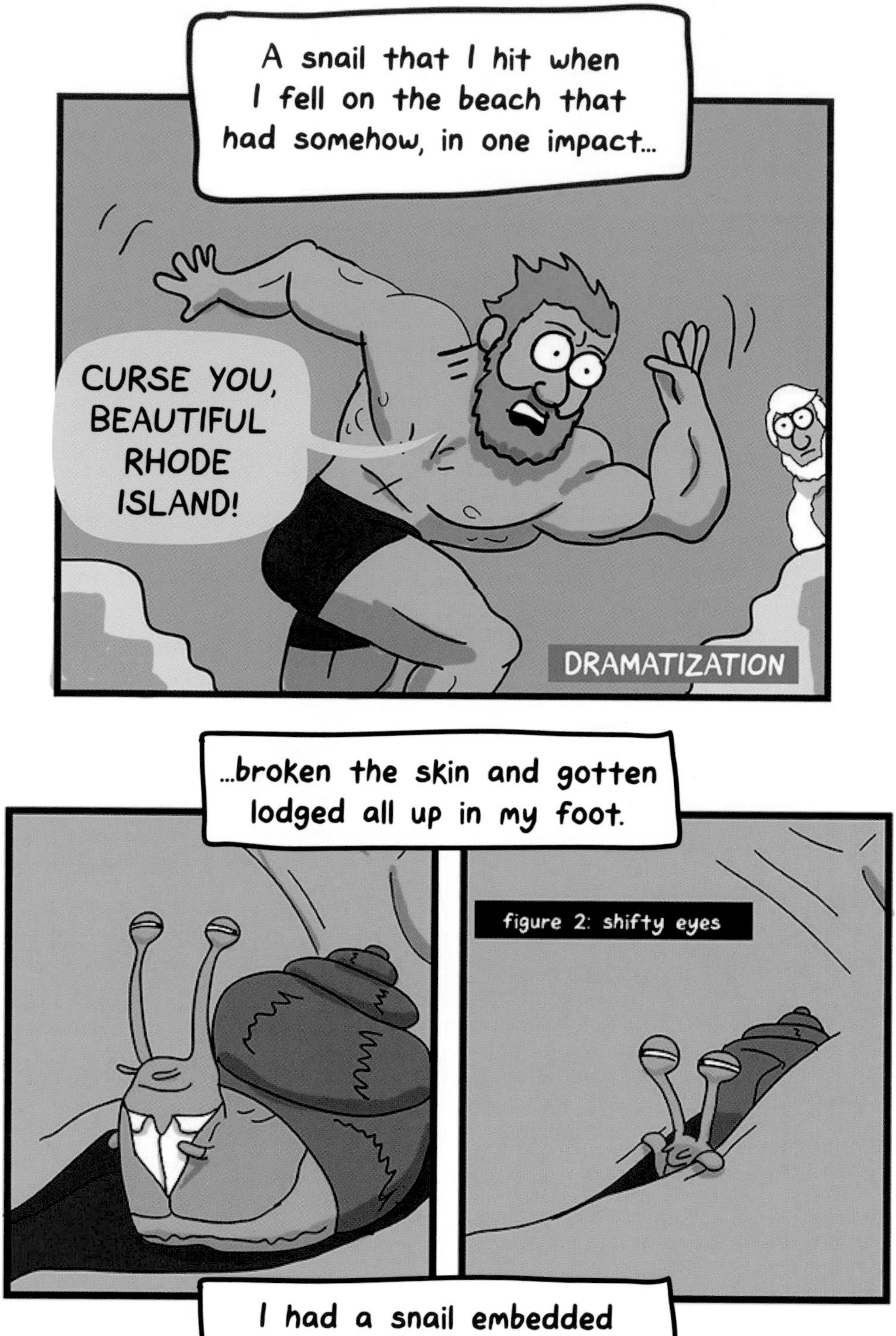
A snail that I hit when I fell on the beach that had somehow, in one impact...
CURSE YOU, BEAUTIFUL RHODE ISLAND!
DRAMATIZATION
...broken the skin and gotten lodged all up in my foot.
figure 2: shifty eyes
I had a snail embedded in my foot.

The PA cut it out with a few short minutes' work, shaking his head and telling me it wasn't actually the first periwinkelectomy he'd performed.

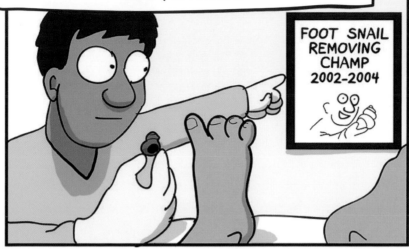

FOOT SNAIL
REMOVING
CHAMP
2002-2004

A couple stitches closed the small wound.

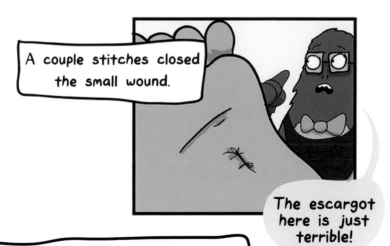

The escargot here is just terrible!

He sent me away with the snail shell and the X-rays, which I still have years and years later.

CHAPTER 2

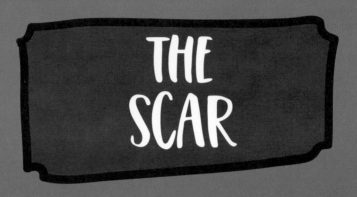

# THE SCAR

told by Anonymous

I do not have
a thyroid anymore
due to benign tumors
that made breathing hard.

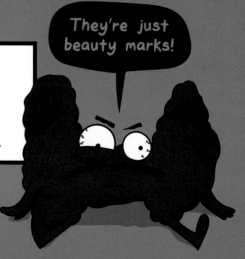

They're just
beauty marks!

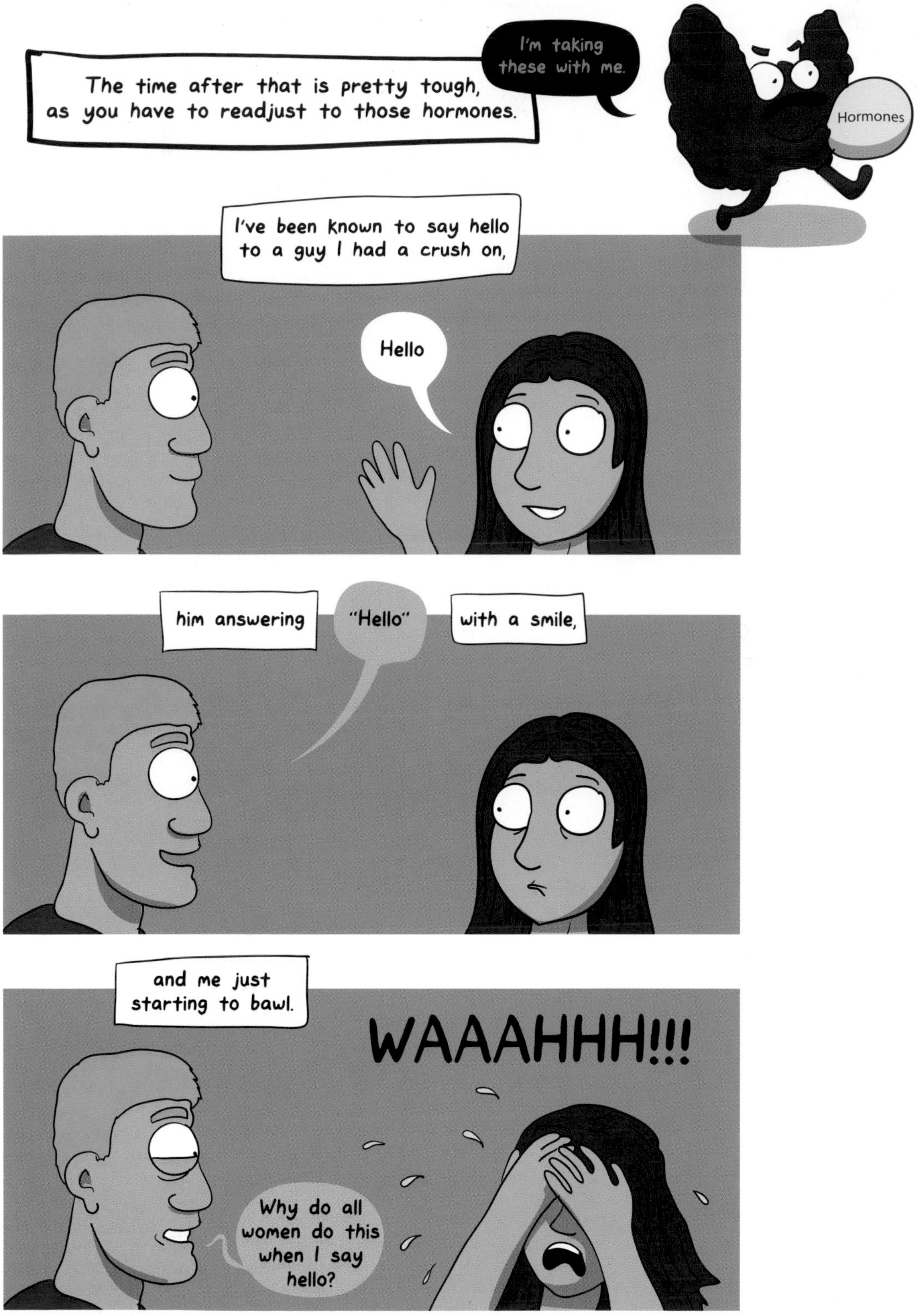
The time after that is pretty tough, as you have to readjust to those hormones.
I'm taking these with me.
Hormones
I've been known to say hello to a guy I had a crush on,
Hello
him answering
"Hello"
with a smile,
and me just starting to bawl.
WAAAHHH!!!
Why do all women do this when I say hello?

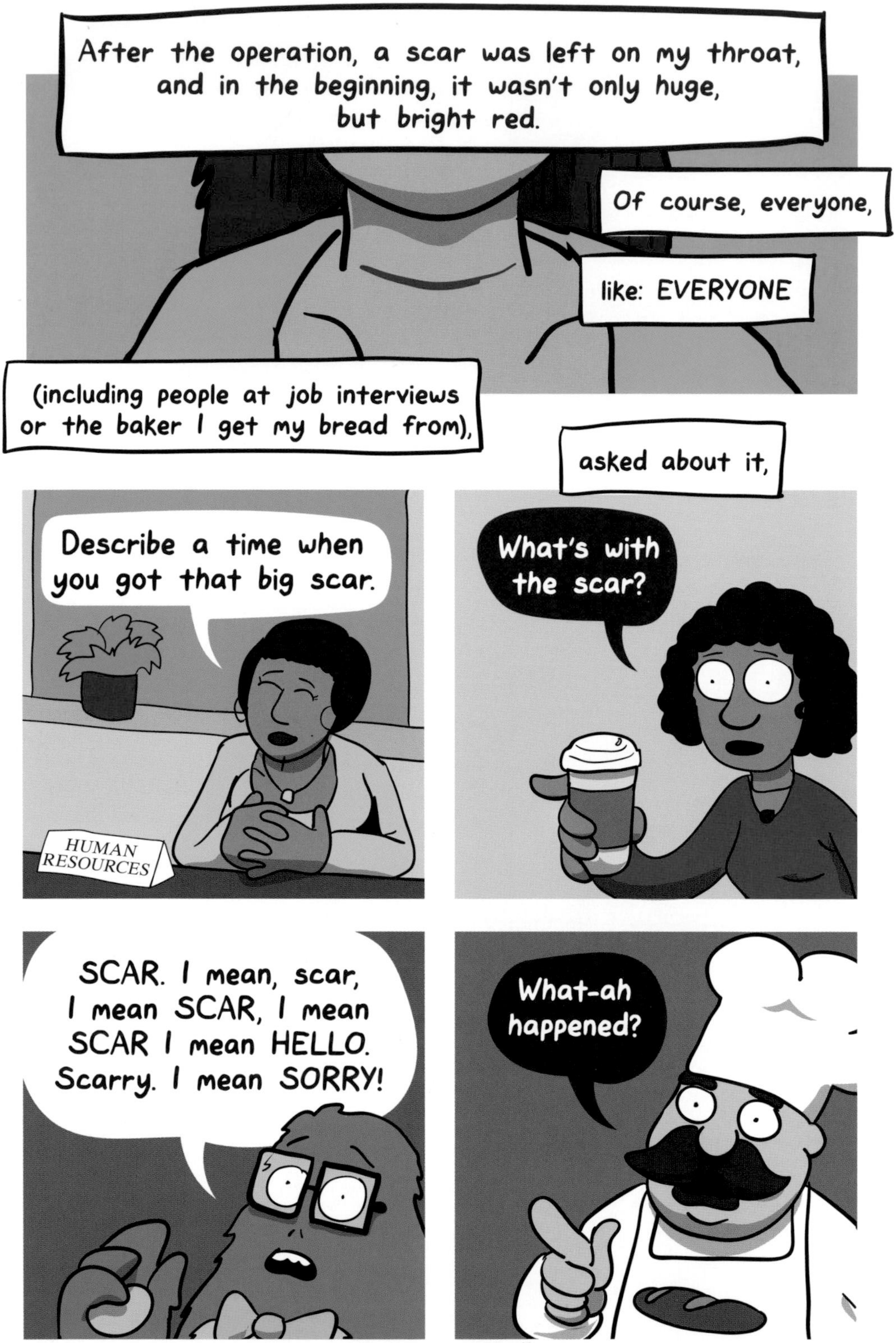
After the operation, a scar was left on my throat, and in the beginning, it wasn't only huge, but bright red.
Of course, everyone,
like: EVERYONE
(including people at job interviews or the baker I get my bread from),
asked about it,
Describe a time when you got that big scar.
HUMAN RESOURCES
What's with the scar?
SCAR. I mean, scar, I mean SCAR, I mean SCAR I mean HELLO. Scarry. I mean SORRY!
What-ah happened?

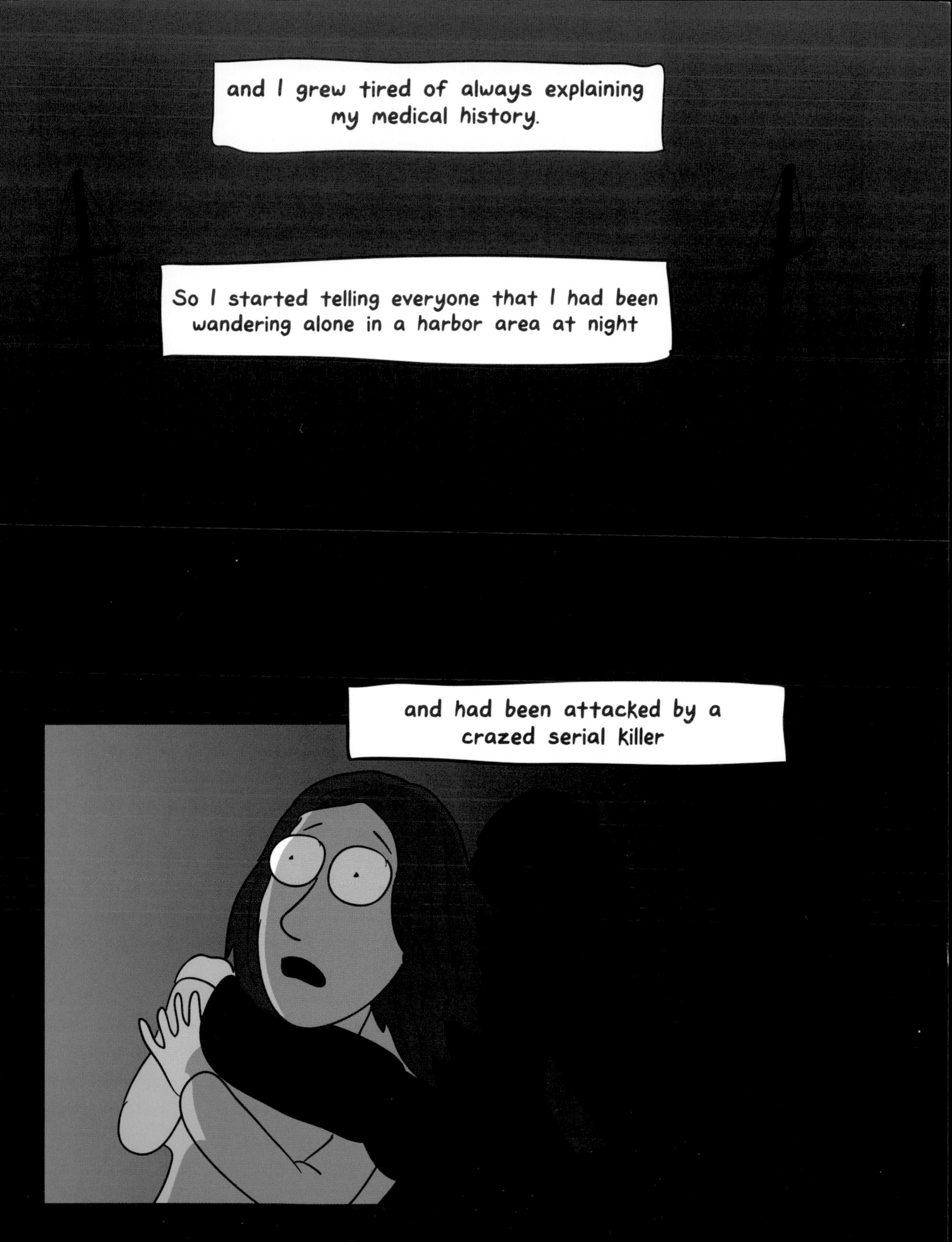
and I grew tired of always explaining my medical history.
So I started telling everyone that I had been wandering alone in a harbor area at night
and had been attacked by a crazed serial killer

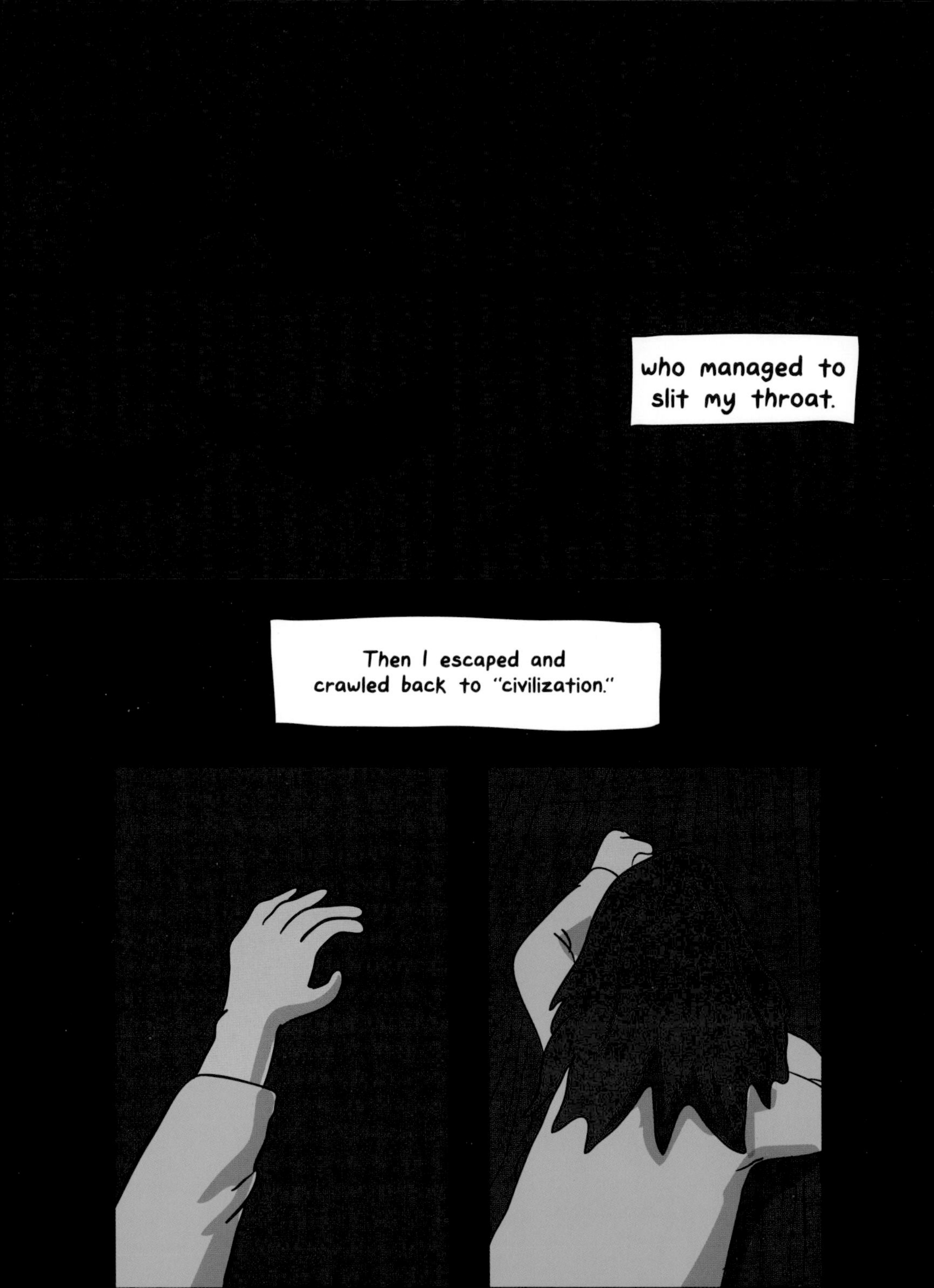
who managed to slit my throat.
Then I escaped and crawled back to "civilization."

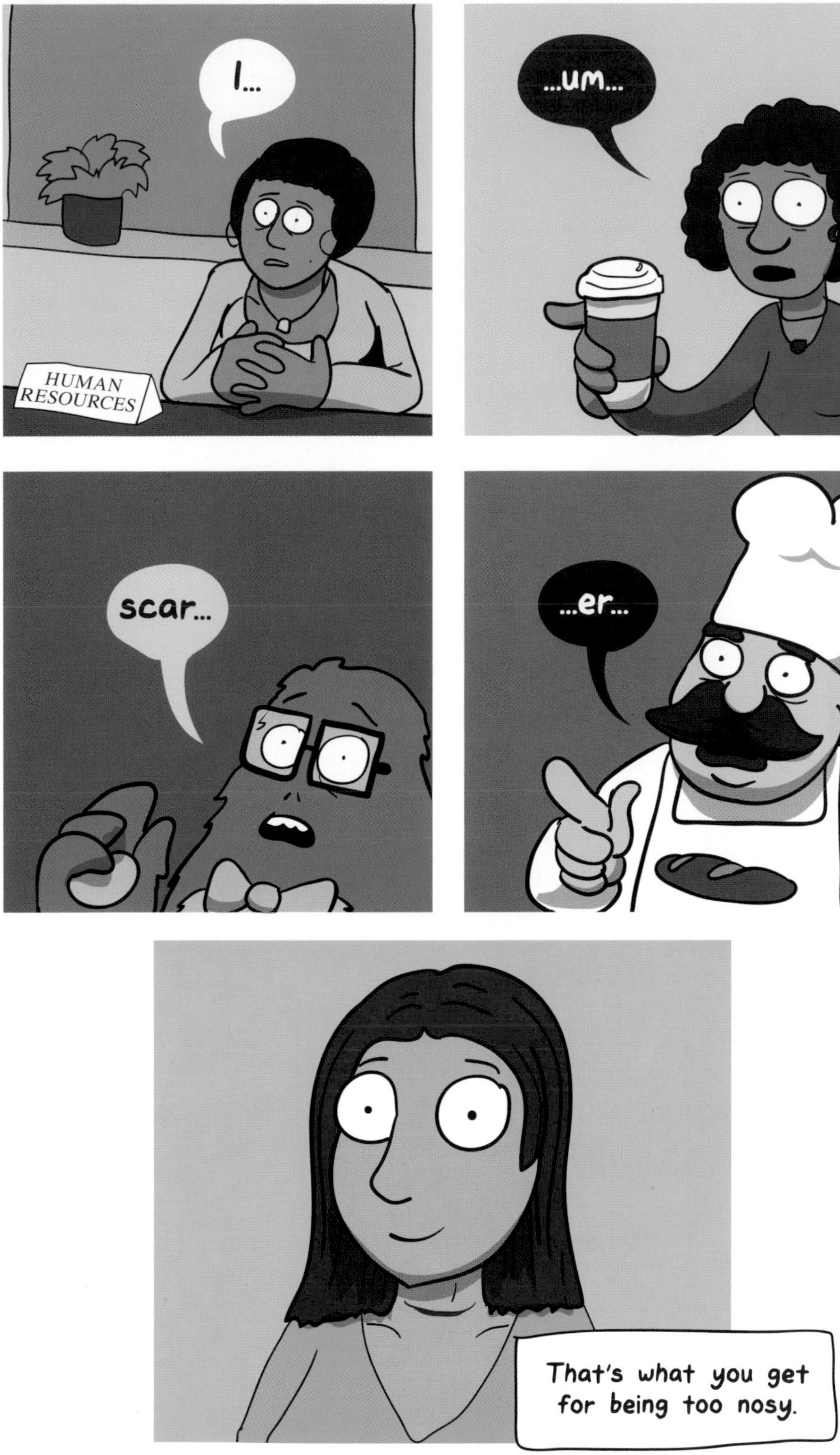
I...
HUMAN RESOURCES
...um...
scar...
...er...
That's what you get for being too nosy.

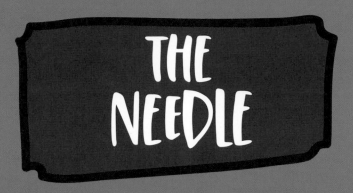

# CHAPTER 3

# THE NEEDLE

told by AR

Back in high school, I took a textiles class.

I hate needles...

We were working on sewing baby quilts.

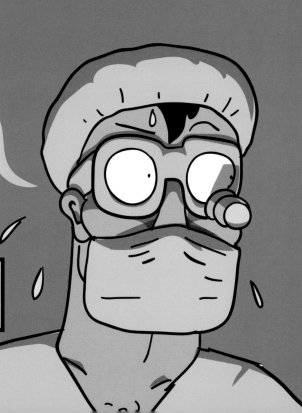

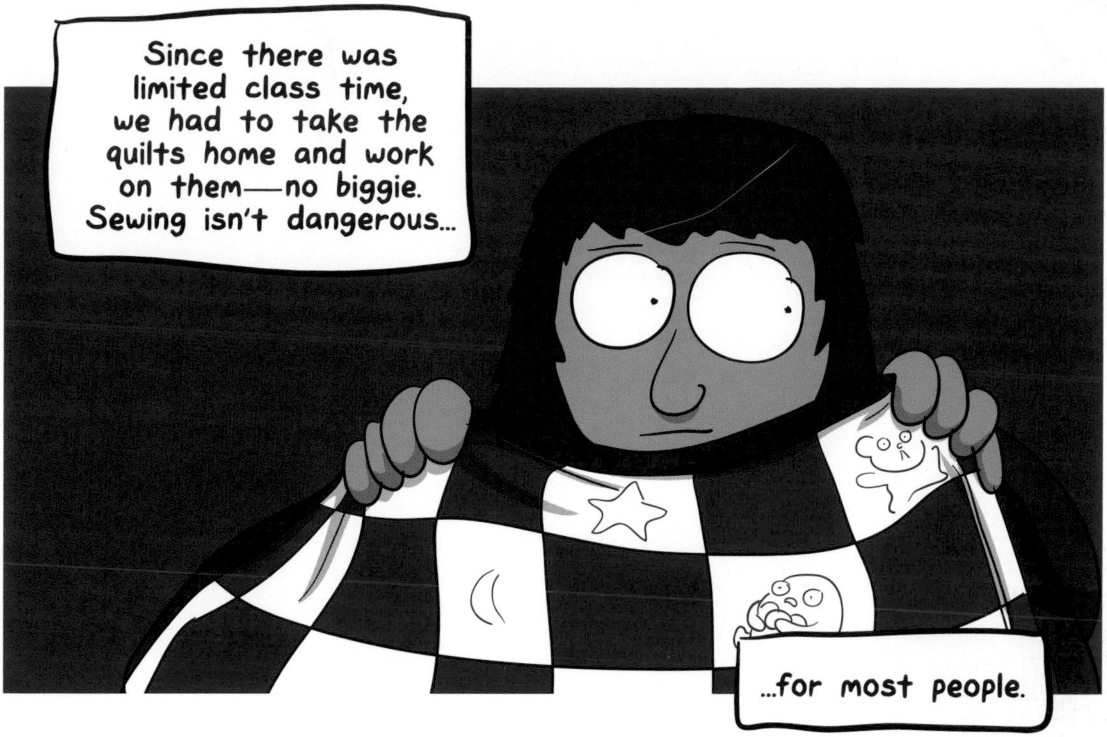
Since there was limited class time, we had to take the quilts home and work on them—no biggie. Sewing isn't dangerous...
...for most people.

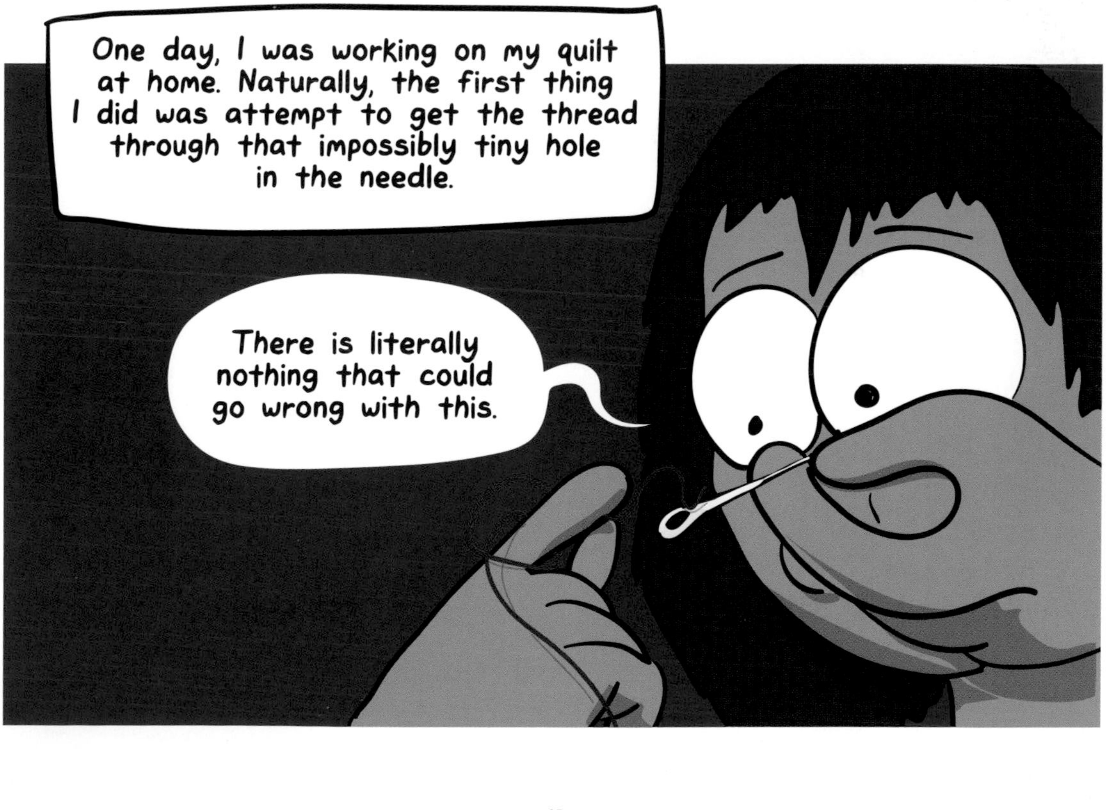
One day, I was working on my quilt at home. Naturally, the first thing I did was attempt to get the thread through that impossibly tiny hole in the needle.
There is literally nothing that could go wrong with this.

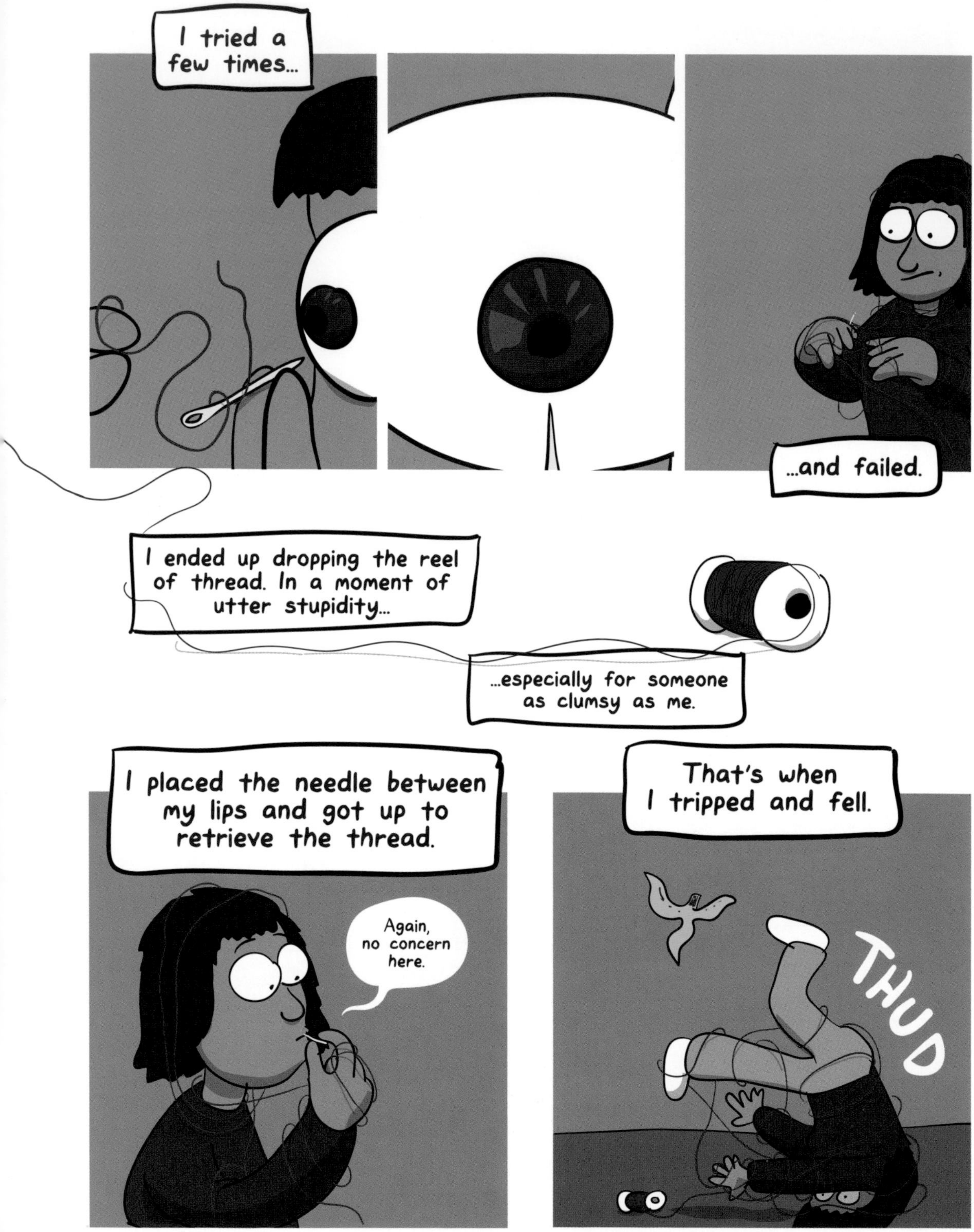
I tried a few times...
...and failed.
I ended up dropping the reel of thread. In a moment of utter stupidity...
...especially for someone as clumsy as me.
I placed the needle between my lips and got up to retrieve the thread.
Again, no concern here.
That's when I tripped and fell.
THUD

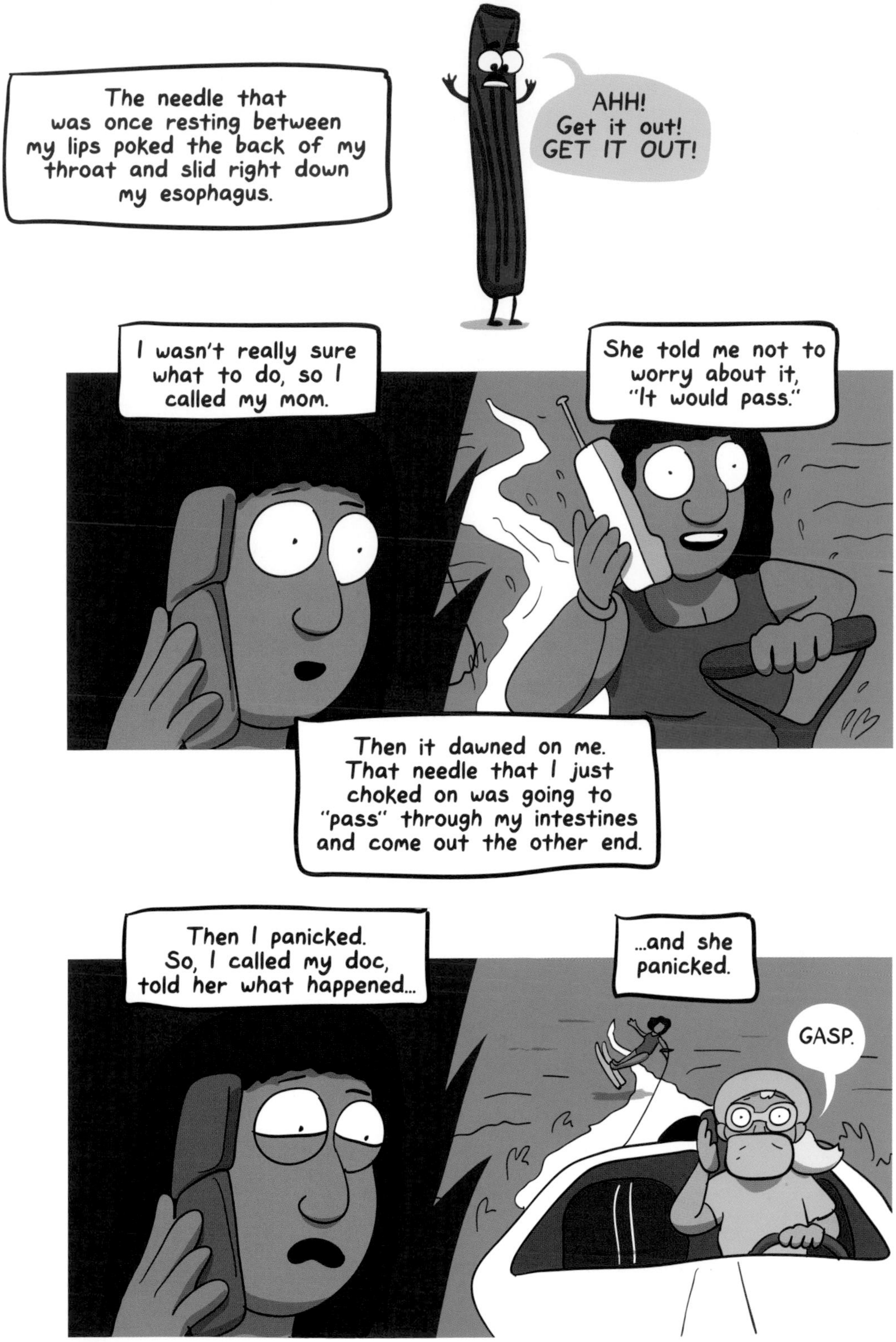
The needle that was once resting between my lips poked the back of my throat and slid right down my esophagus.
AHH! Get it out! GET IT OUT!
I wasn't really sure what to do, so I called my mom.
She told me not to worry about it, "It would pass."
Then it dawned on me. That needle that I just choked on was going to "pass" through my intestines and come out the other end.
Then I panicked. So, I called my doc, told her what happened...
...and she panicked.
GASP.

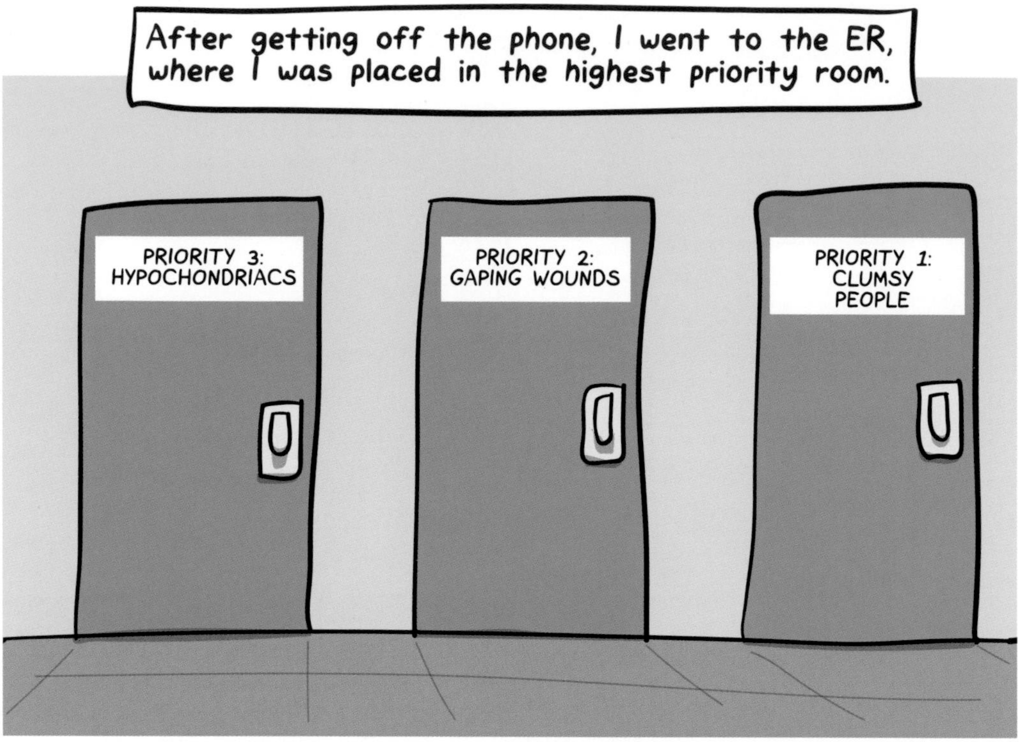
After getting off the phone, I went to the ER, where I was placed in the highest priority room.
PRIORITY 3: HYPOCHONDRIACS
PRIORITY 2: GAPING WOUNDS
PRIORITY 1: CLUMSY PEOPLE

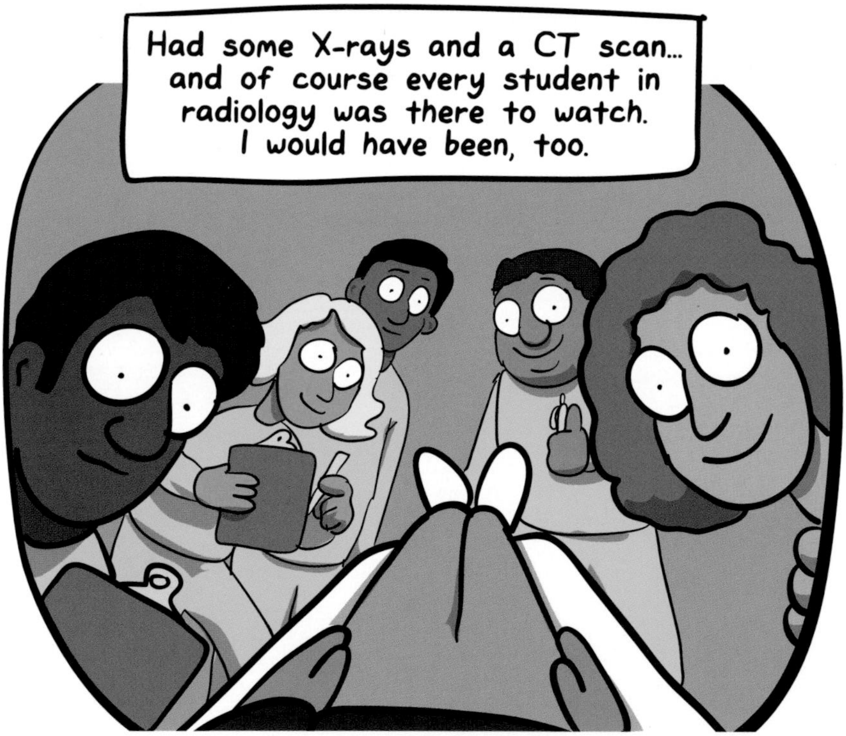
Had some X-rays and a CT scan... and of course every student in radiology was there to watch. I would have been, too.

The CT showed the needle lodged halfway through the side of my duodenum...

You need to keep better digestive TRACT of your needles!

Get it? TRACT?!

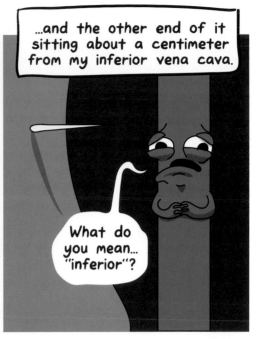

...and the other end of it sitting about a centimeter from my inferior vena cava.

What do you mean... "inferior"?

This caused a lot of panic in the ER.

They sent me straight to surgery. I ended up having an endoscopy to remove the needle.

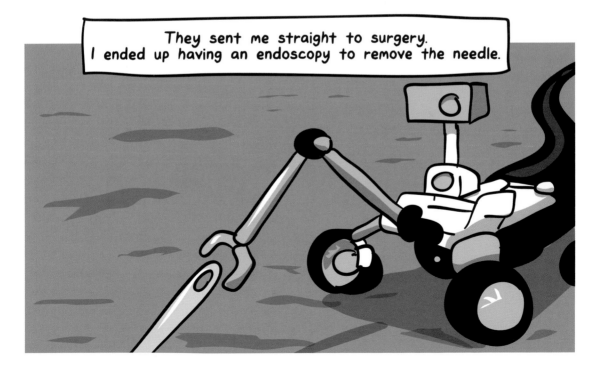

The surgeon said I was lucky it was in the duodenum because otherwise they would have had to do a much more invasive surgery. Turns out those scopes only go so far.

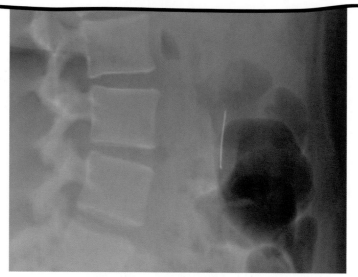

(Actual X-ray)

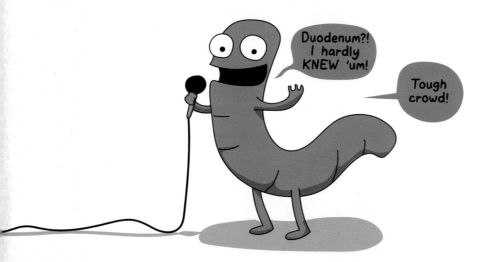

Duodenum?! I hardly KNEW 'um!

Tough crowd!

CHAPTER 4

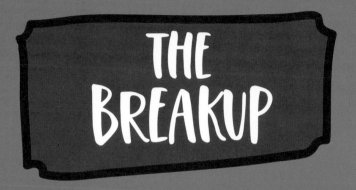

THE
BREAKUP

told by Funkstonian

I recently went through
a very horrible breakup.

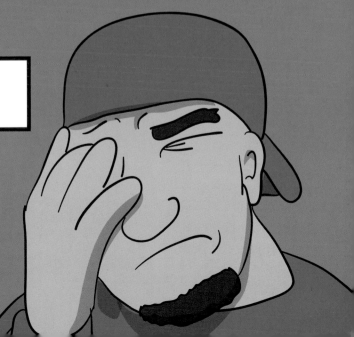

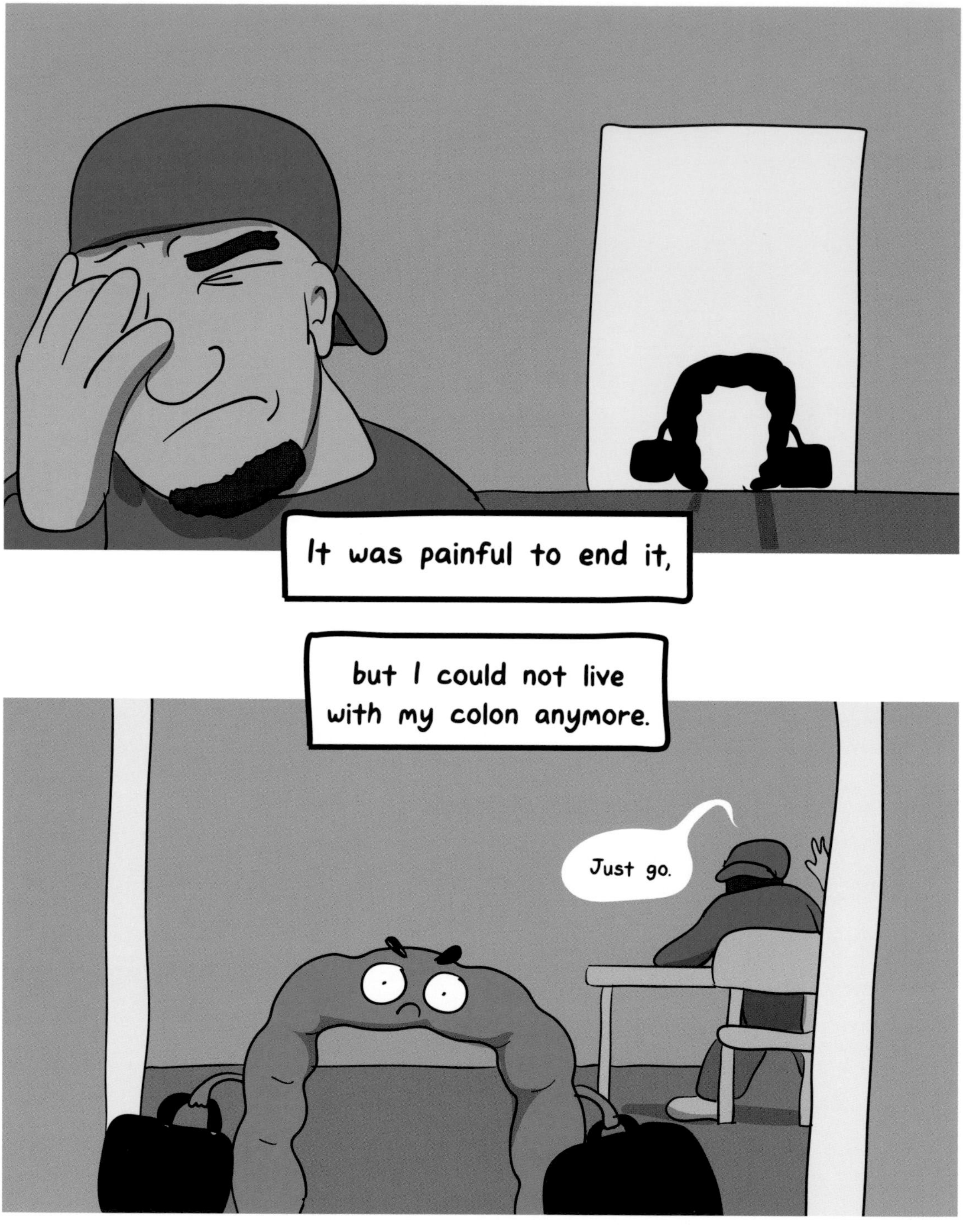
It was painful to end it,
but I could not live with my colon anymore.
Just go.

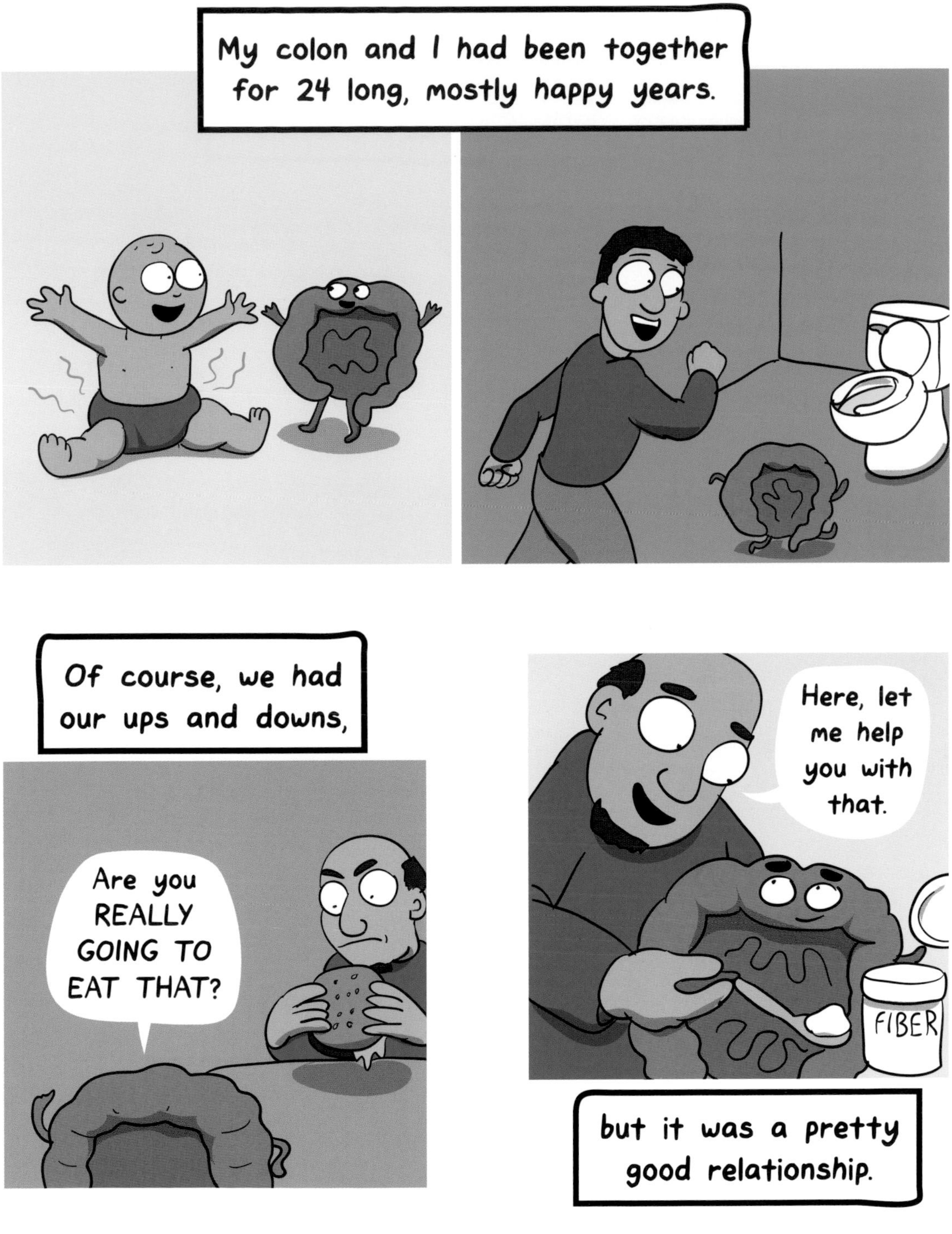
My colon and I had been together for 24 long, mostly happy years.
Of course, we had our ups and downs,
Are you REALLY GOING TO EAT THAT?
Here, let me help you with that.
FIBER
but it was a pretty good relationship.

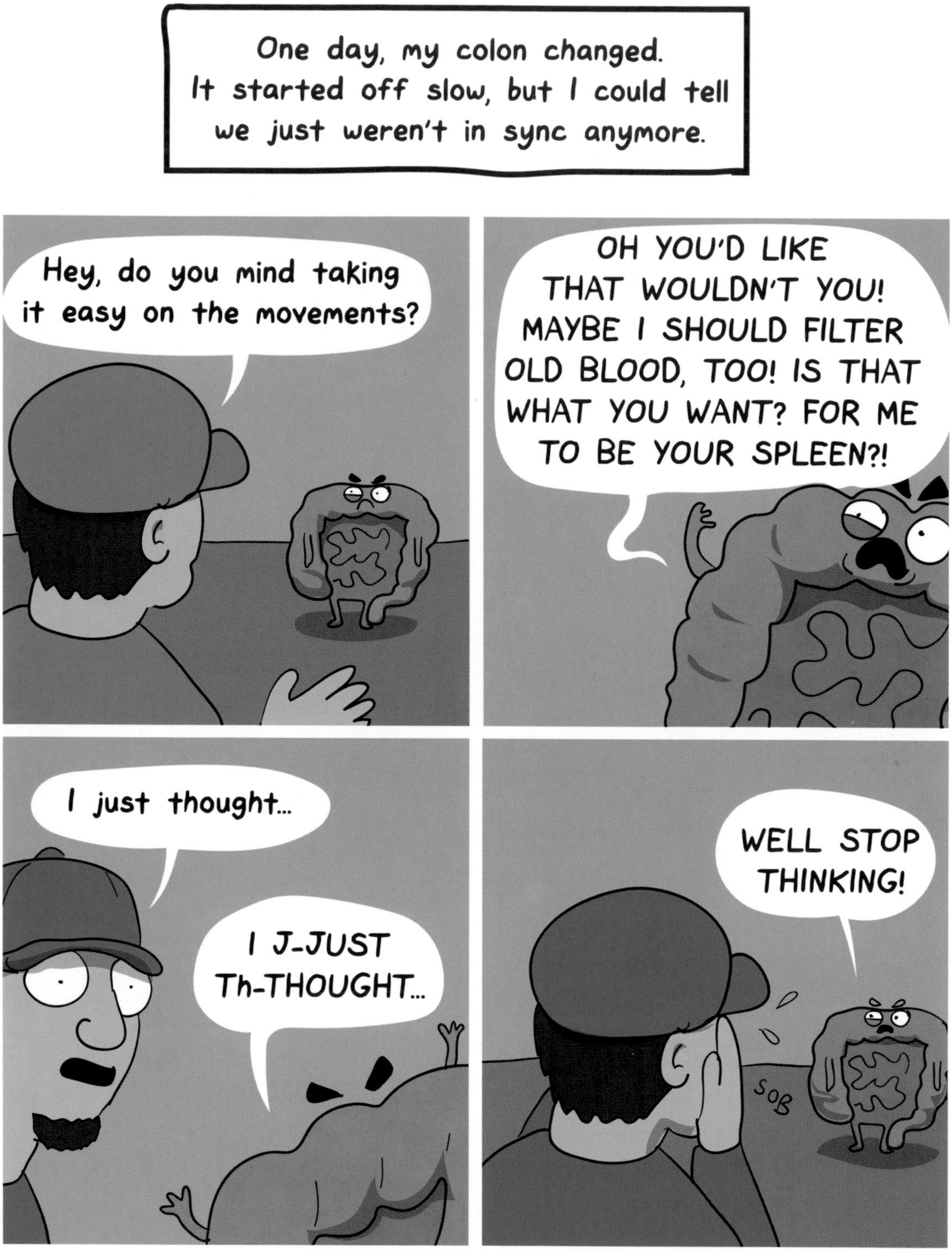
One day, my colon changed. It started off slow, but I could tell we just weren't in sync anymore.
Hey, do you mind taking it easy on the movements?
OH YOU'D LIKE THAT WOULDN'T YOU! MAYBE I SHOULD FILTER OLD BLOOD, TOO! IS THAT WHAT YOU WANT? FOR ME TO BE YOUR SPLEEN?!
I just thought...
I J-JUST Th-THOUGHT...
WELL STOP THINKING!
SOB

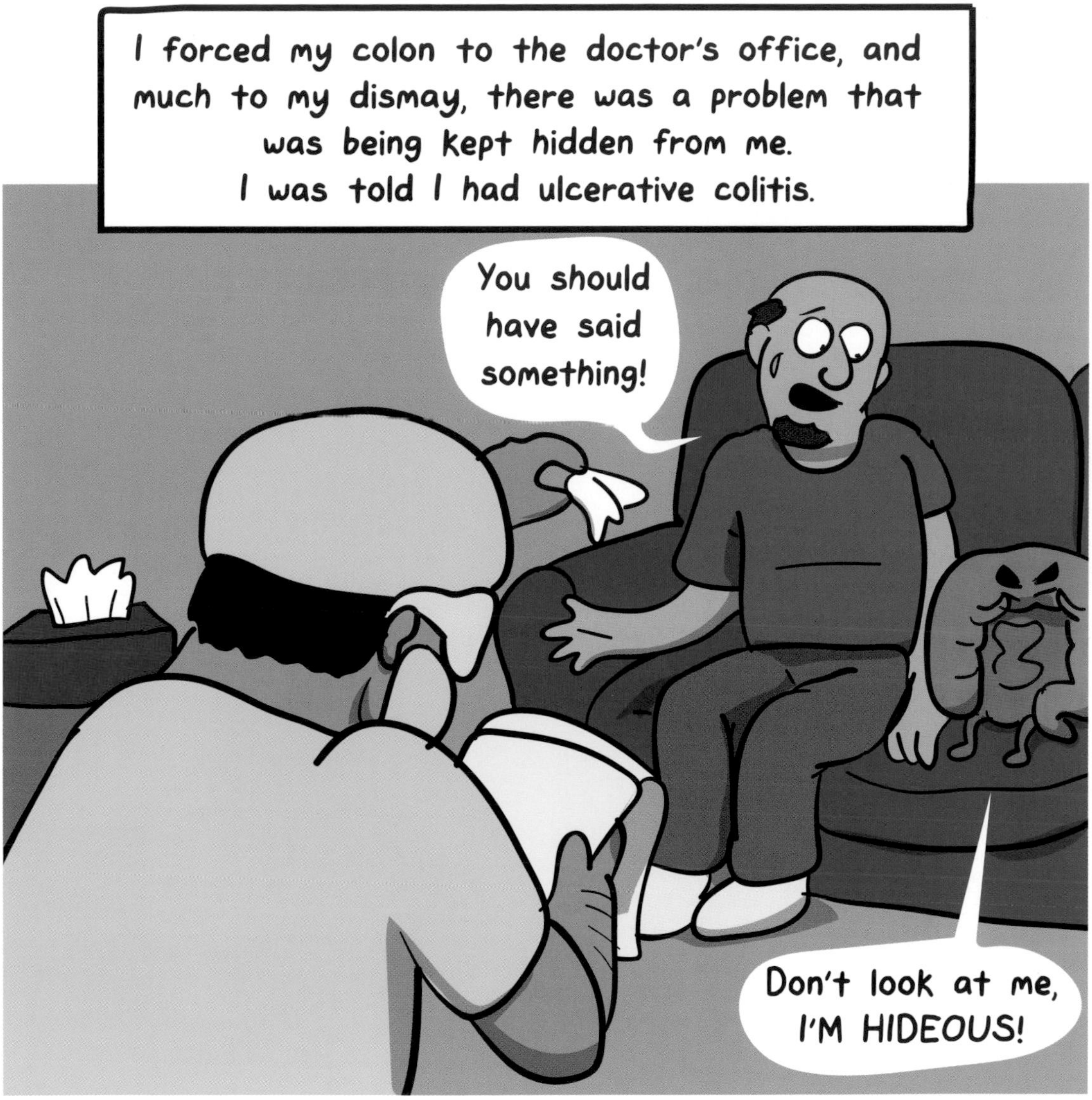
I forced my colon to the doctor's office, and much to my dismay, there was a problem that was being kept hidden from me. I was told I had ulcerative colitis.
You should have said something!
Don't look at me, I'M HIDEOUS!

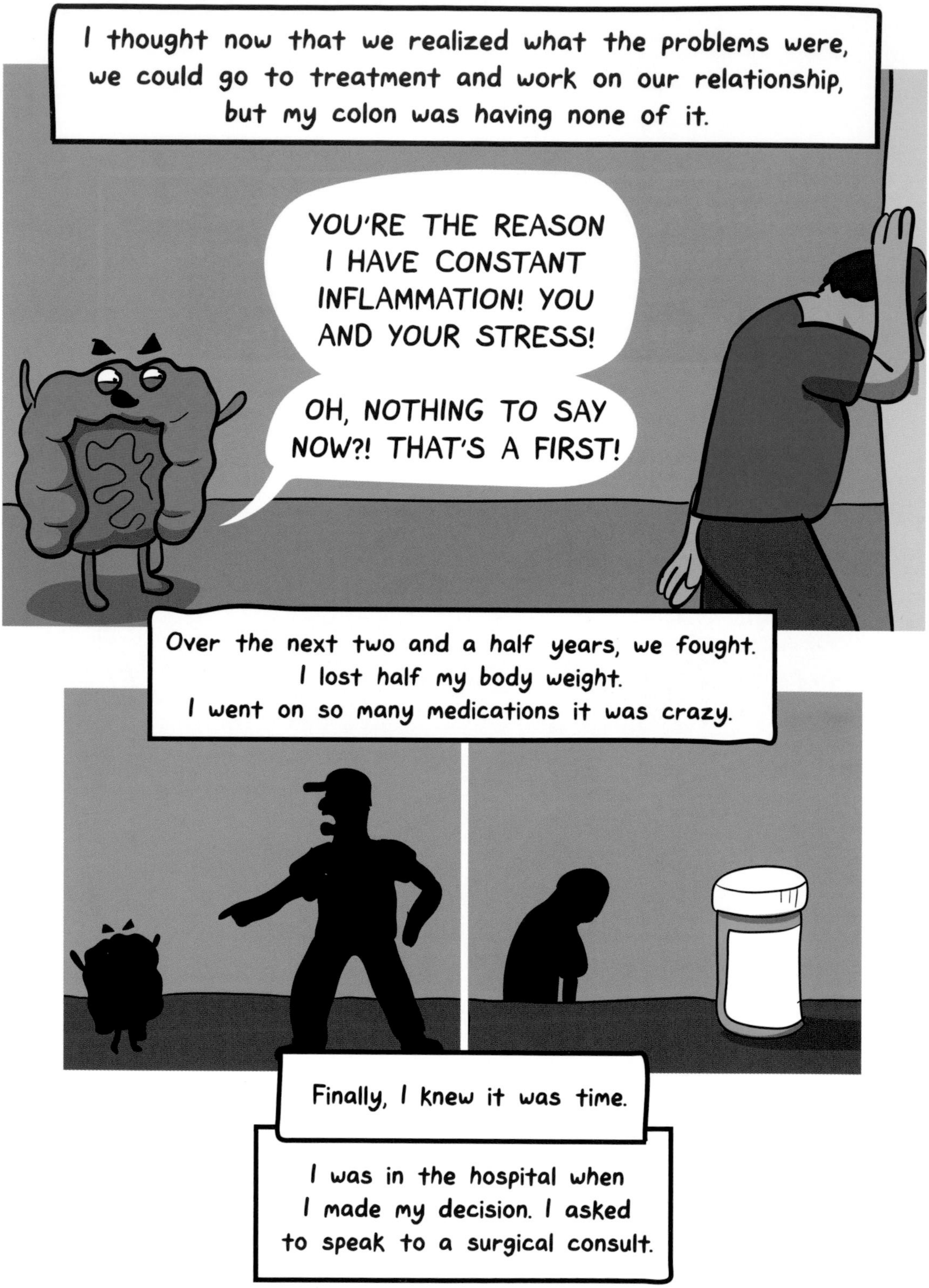
I thought now that we realized what the problems were, we could go to treatment and work on our relationship, but my colon was having none of it.
YOU'RE THE REASON I HAVE CONSTANT INFLAMMATION! YOU AND YOUR STRESS!
OH, NOTHING TO SAY NOW?! THAT'S A FIRST!
Over the next two and a half years, we fought. I lost half my body weight. I went on so many medications it was crazy.
Finally, I knew it was time.
I was in the hospital when I made my decision. I asked to speak to a surgical consult.

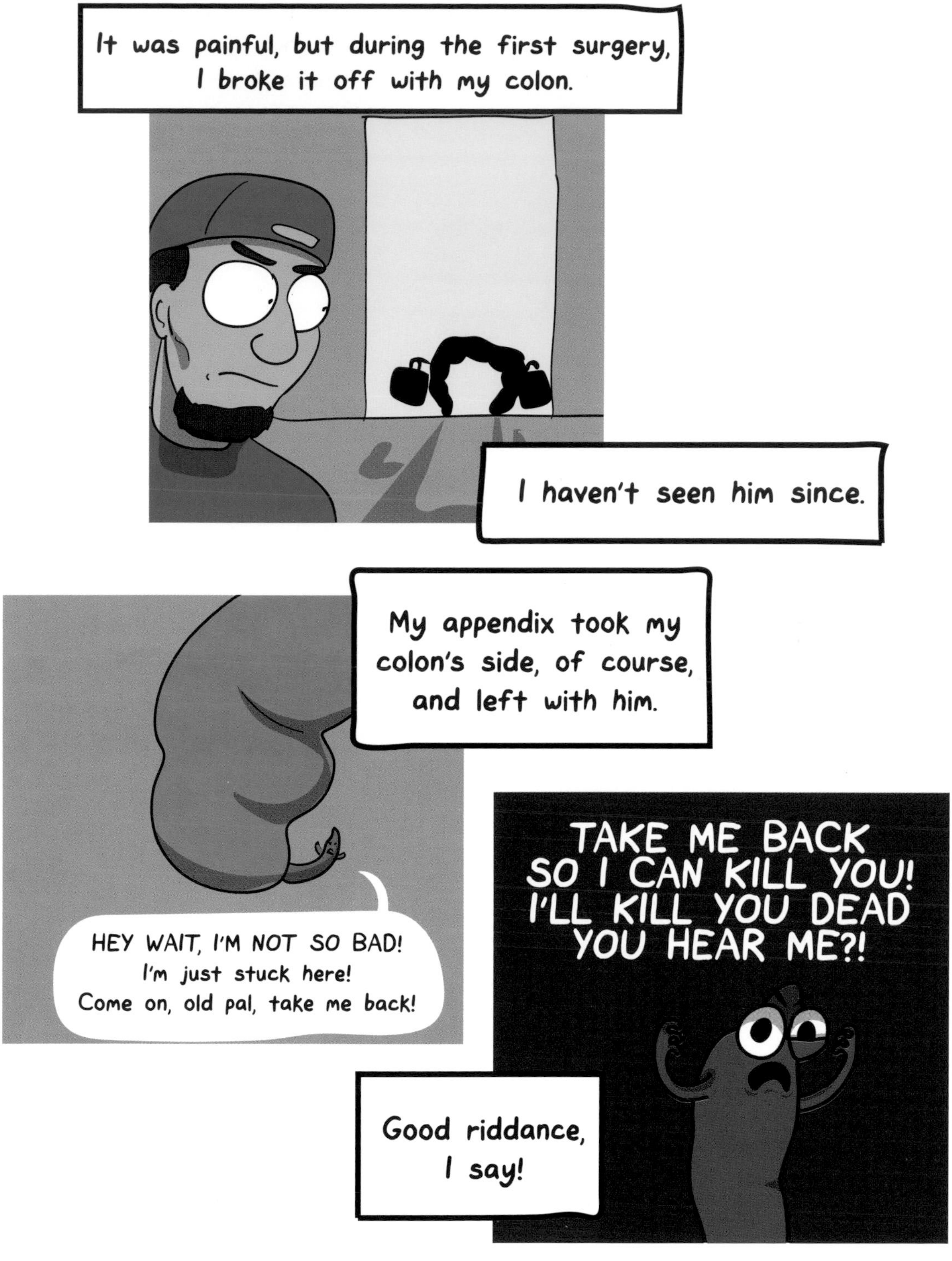
It was painful, but during the first surgery, I broke it off with my colon.
I haven't seen him since.
My appendix took my colon's side, of course, and left with him.
HEY WAIT, I'M NOT SO BAD! I'm just stuck here! Come on, old pal, take me back!
TAKE ME BACK SO I CAN KILL YOU! I'LL KILL YOU DEAD YOU HEAR ME?!
Good riddance, I say!

My small intestine was there for me through the entire thing. In fact, during the second surgery, it offered to take my colon's place as a J-pouch.

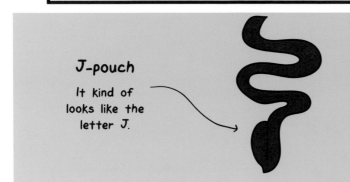

J-pouch
It kind of looks like the letter J.
When an entire colon (aka, the large intestine) is removed, the small intestine can be reattached to the "exit" with a small reservoir.
It allows the patient to do his or her business pretty normally without using an external bag.

I couldn't have made it through without the proper support and love of my small intestine. During the third and final surgery, we will be making the change permanent.

We should also consider putting that on the INSIDE of your body.

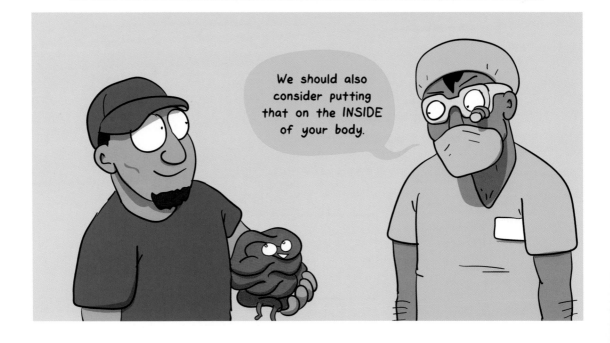

I am very happy now.
I finally realize that it is
not necessarily about the quantity,
but rather the quality of organs that matter.

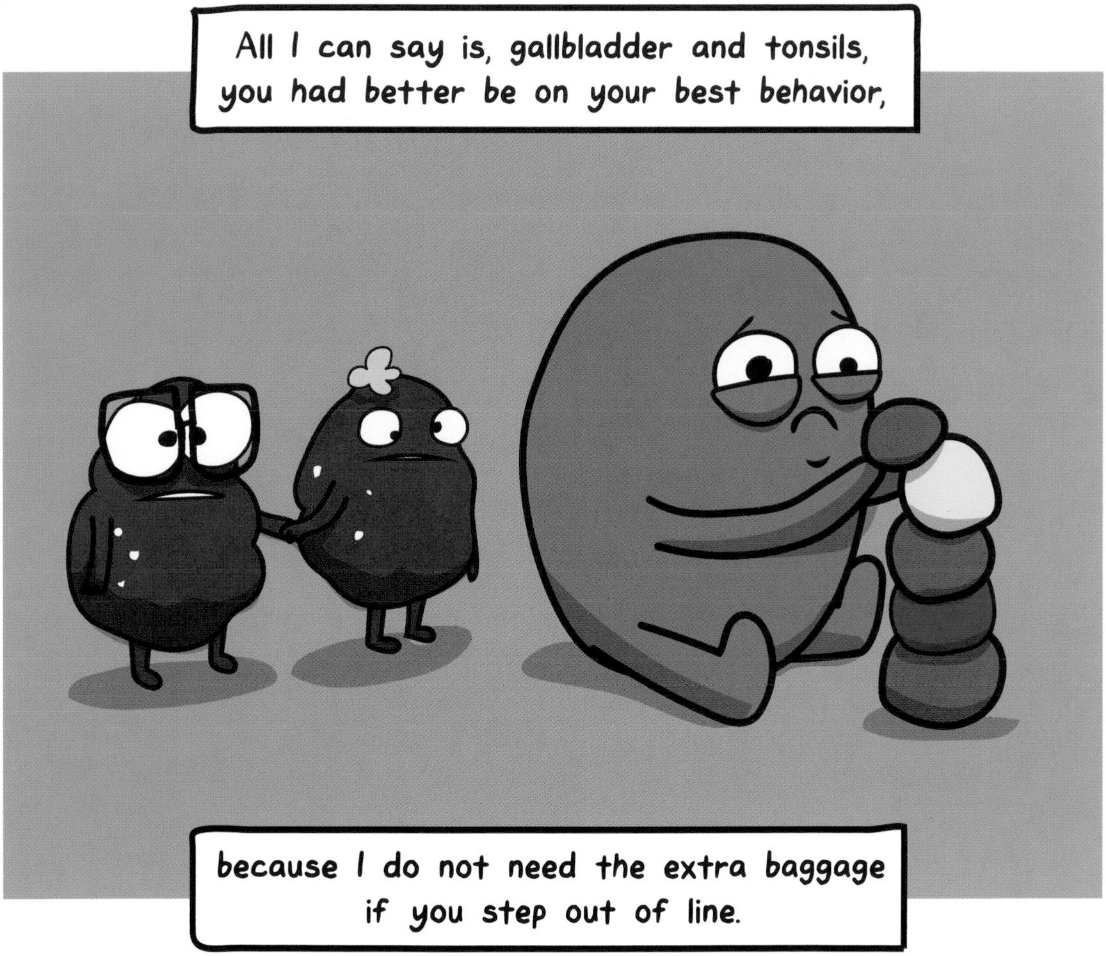
All I can say is, gallbladder and tonsils, you had better be on your best behavior,
because I do not need the extra baggage if you step out of line.

CHAPTER 5

# THE BATTLE

told by Sarah Flanigan

Come on! We've got butterflies to catch!

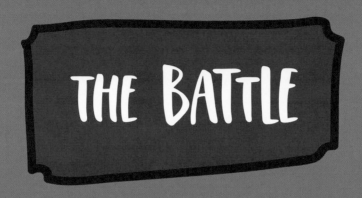

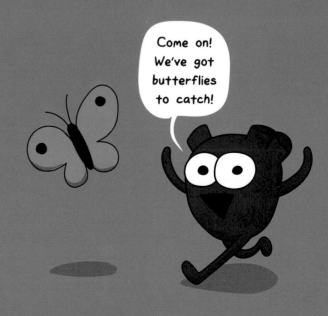

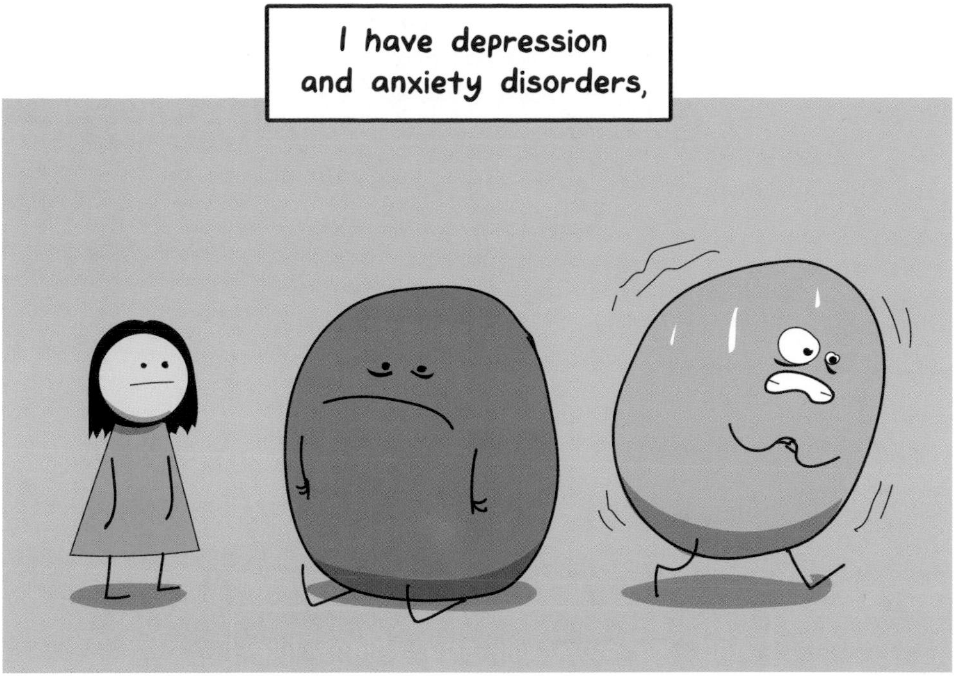
I have depression
and anxiety disorders,

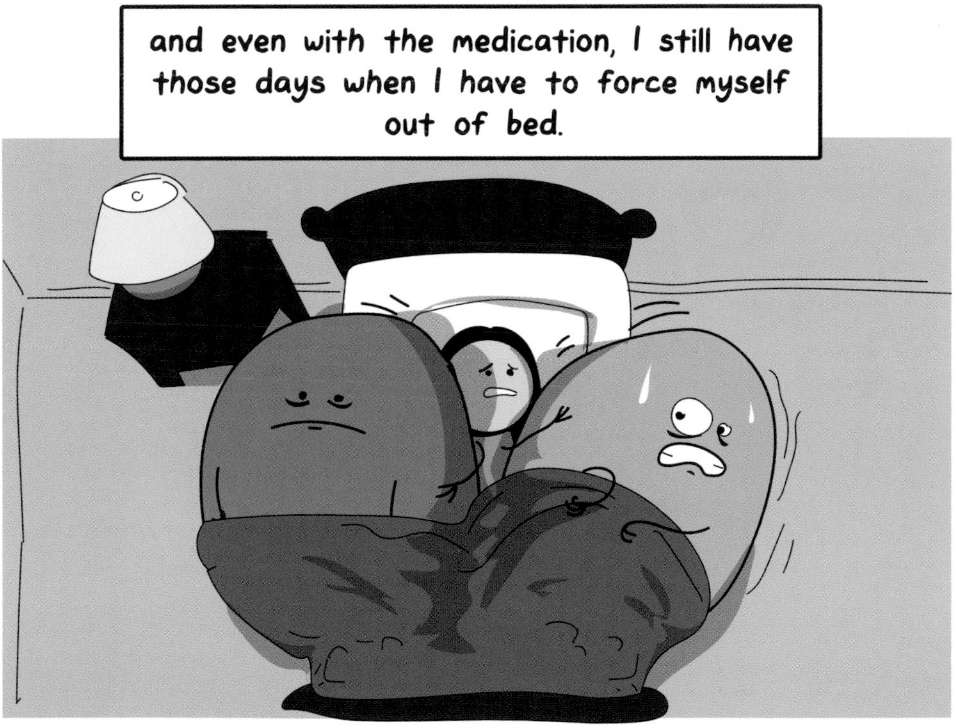
and even with the medication, I still have
those days when I have to force myself
out of bed.

And I can't rally the energy or motivation to do anything.

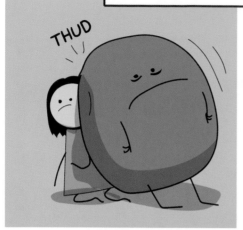

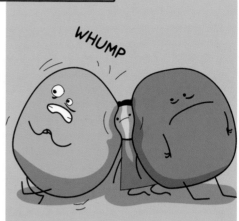

And, my mom will say things like,

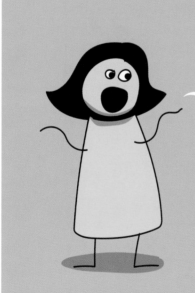

"You were so happy and energetic yesterday, you got so much done."

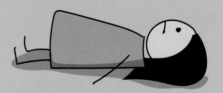

(It makes me cringe to just think about her saying that.)

So I told her this:
Depression and anxiety are teammates
and I'm the opposing team.

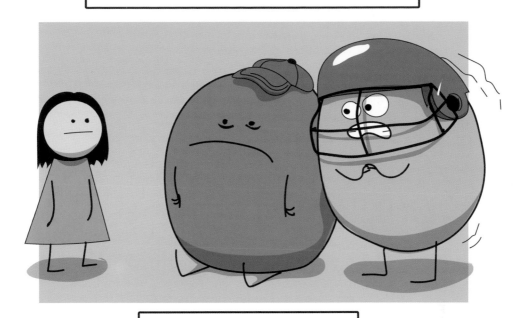

Their one and only goal
is to drag me down.

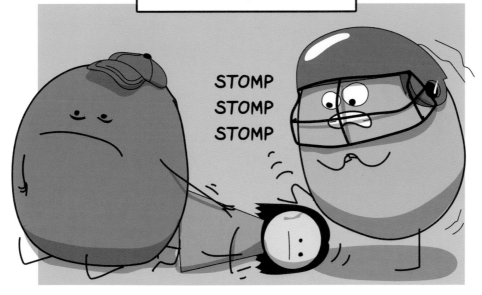

STOMP
STOMP
STOMP

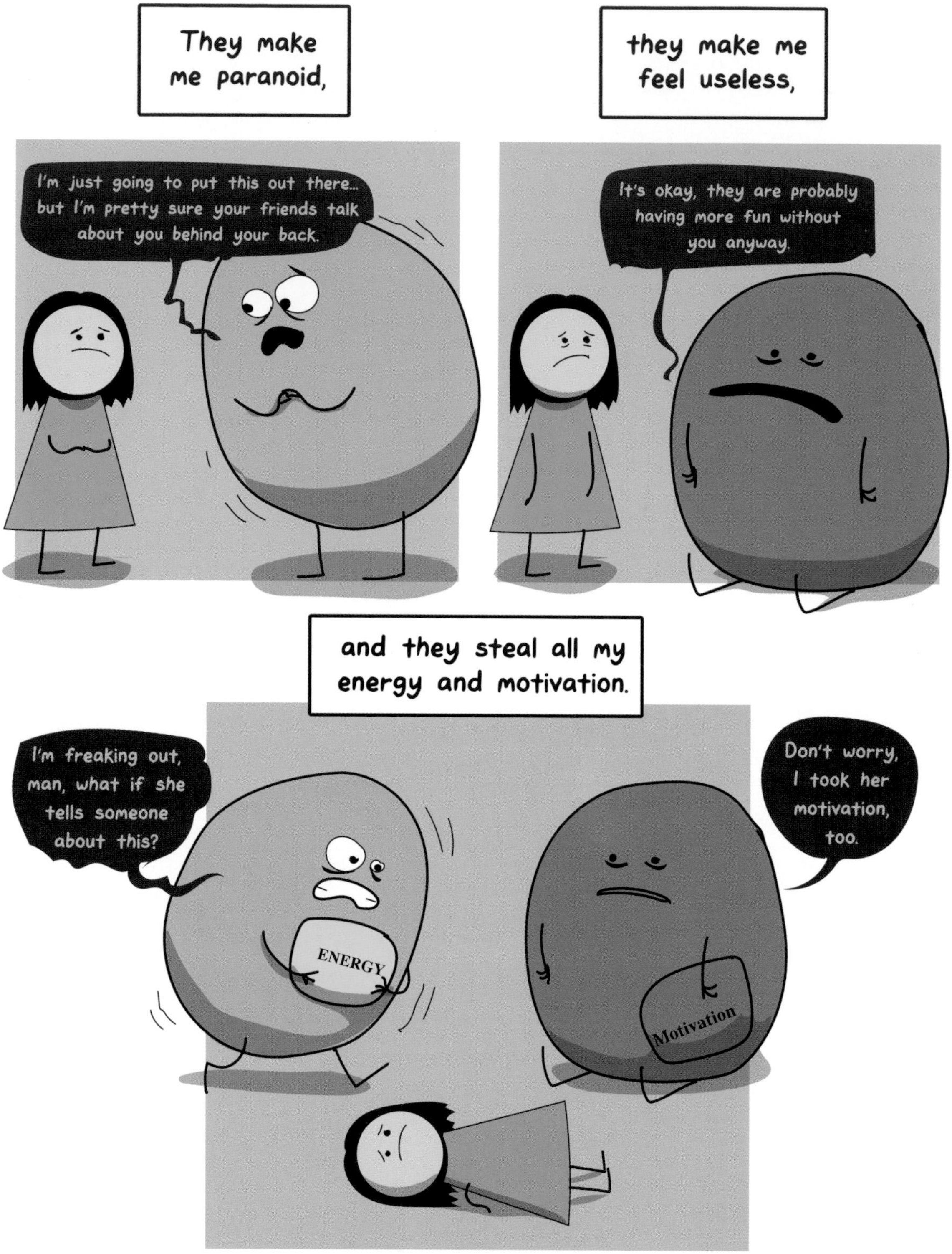
They make me paranoid,
I'm just going to put this out there... but I'm pretty sure your friends talk about you behind your back.
they make me feel useless,
It's okay, they are probably having more fun without you anyway.
and they steal all my energy and motivation.
I'm freaking out, man, what if she tells someone about this?
ENERGY
Don't worry, I took her motivation, too.
Motivation

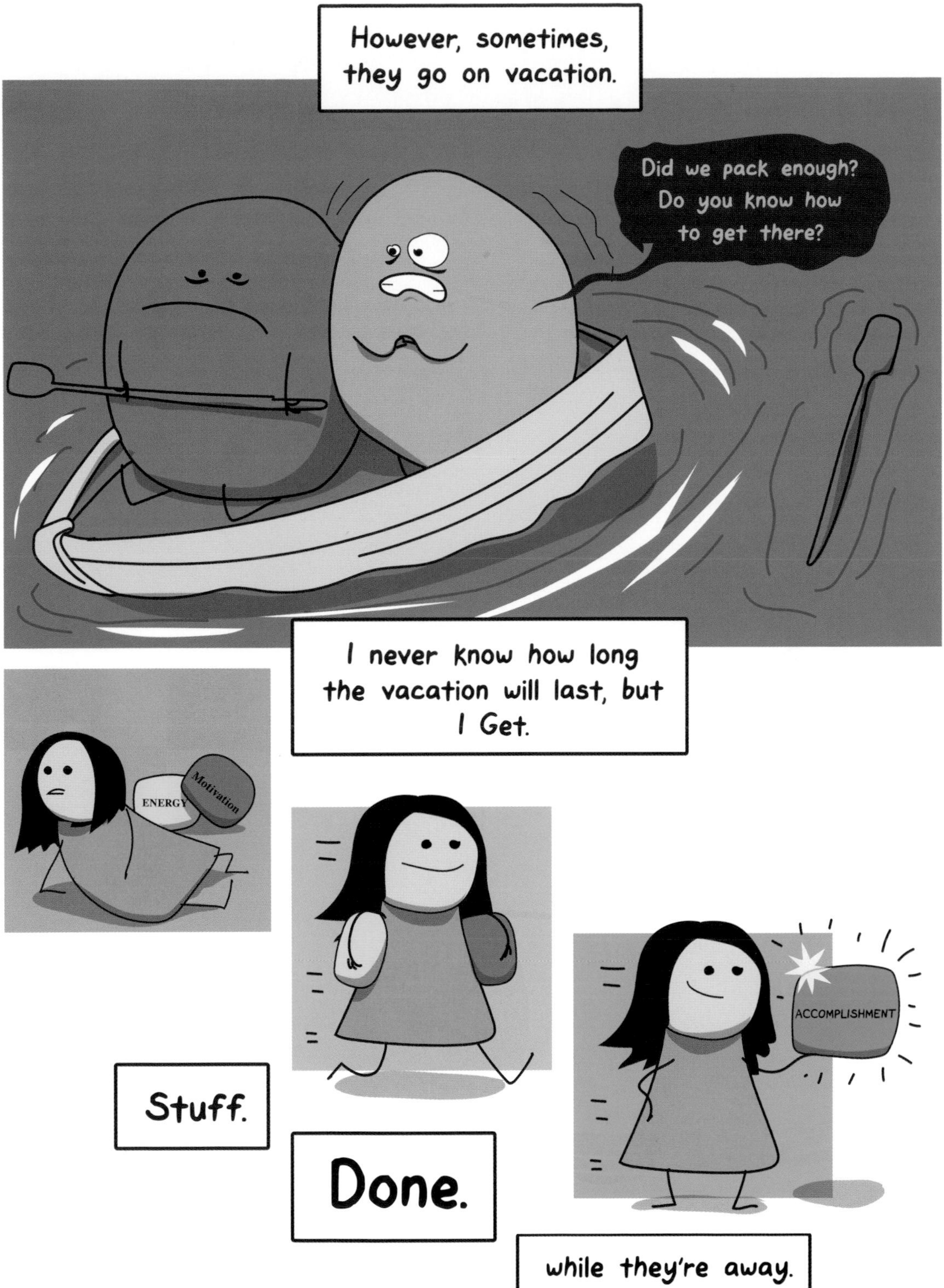
However, sometimes, they go on vacation.
Did we pack enough? Do you know how to get there?
I never know how long the vacation will last, but I Get.
ENERGY
Motivation
Stuff.
Done.
ACCOMPLISHMENT
while they're away.

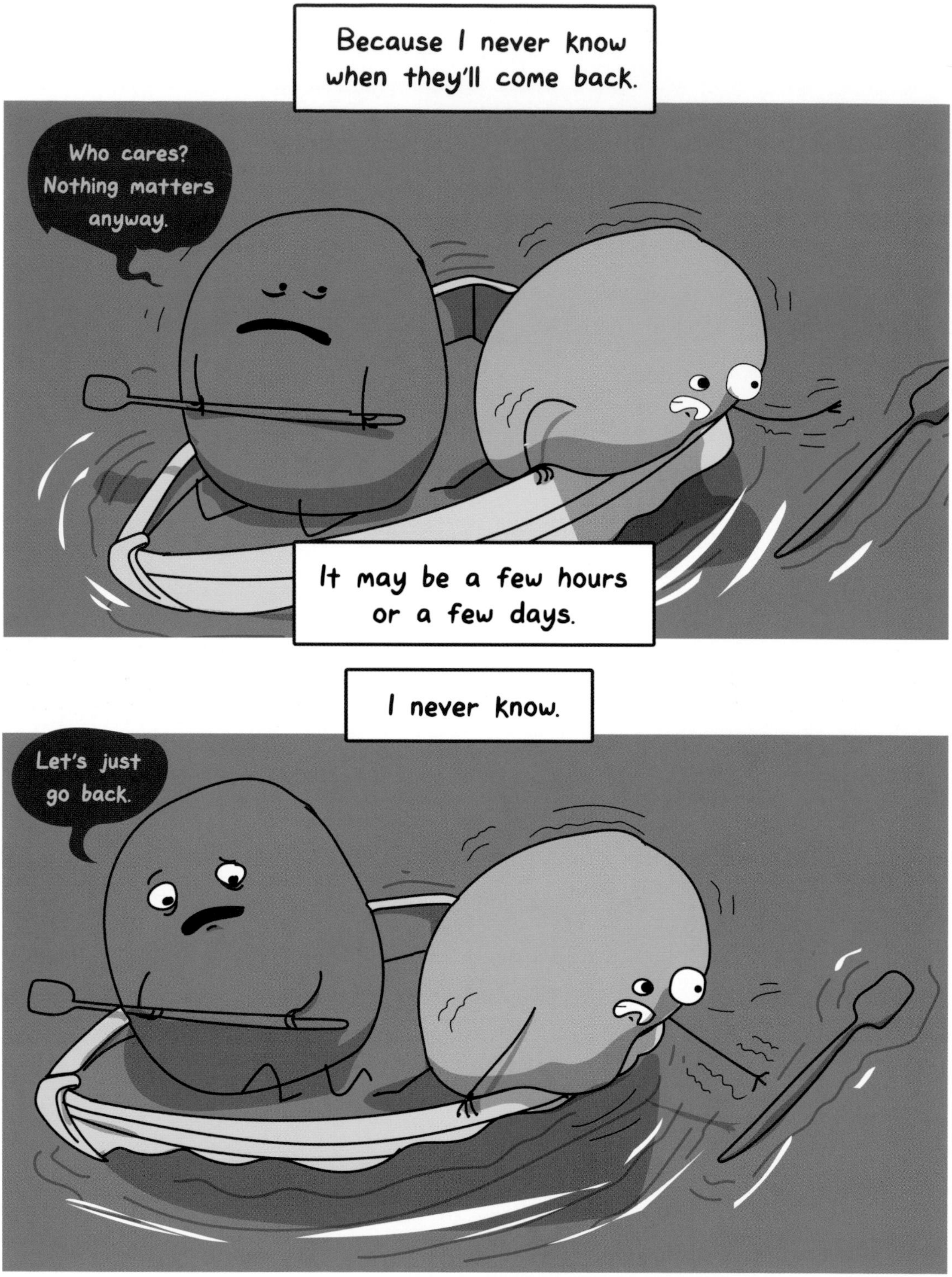
Because I never know when they'll come back.
Who cares? Nothing matters anyway.
It may be a few hours or a few days.
I never know.
Let's just go back.

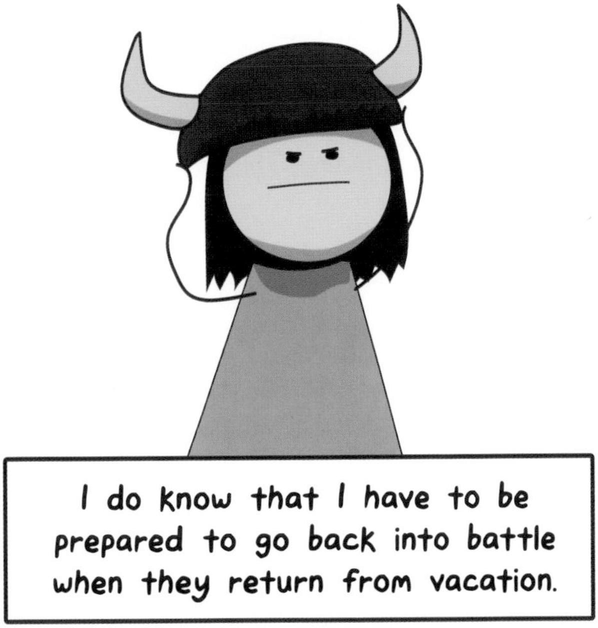
I do know that I have to be prepared to go back into battle when they return from vacation.

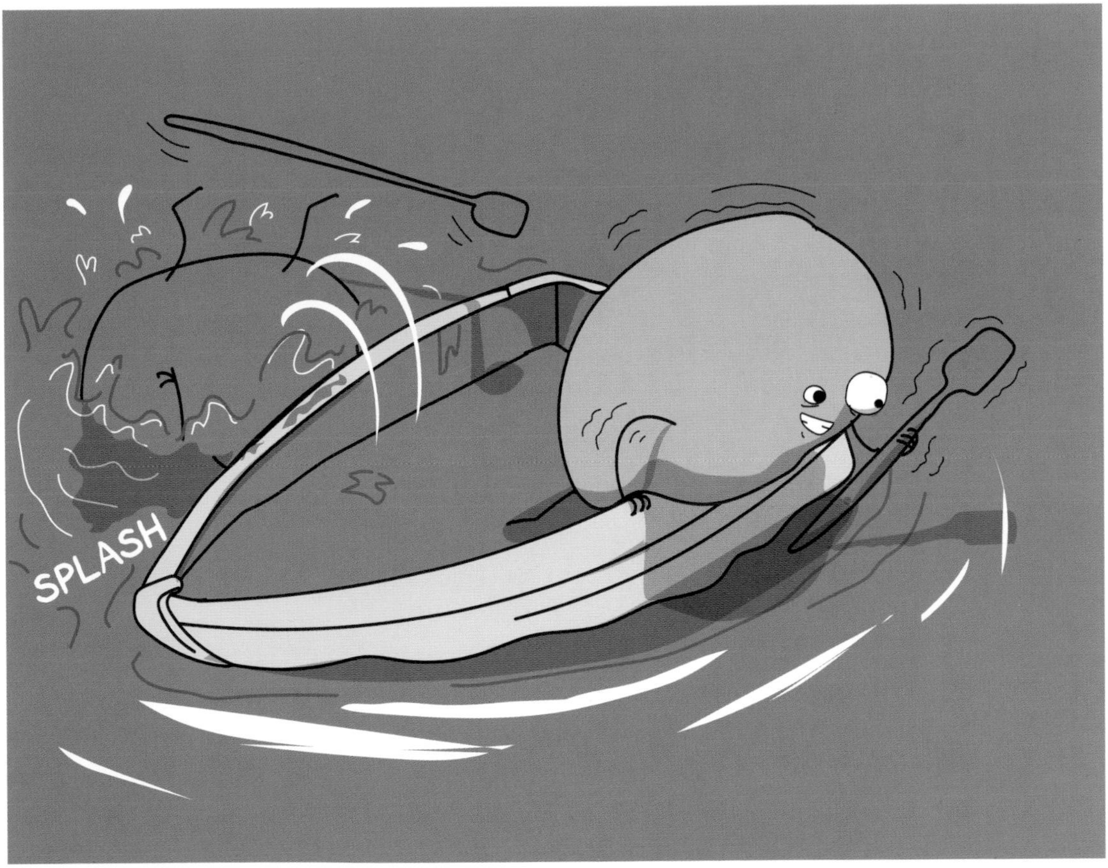
SPLASH

CHAPTER 6

# APPENDICITIS?

told by Josh Cecil

NURSE! THIS MAN'S TUMMY IS OUCHY!

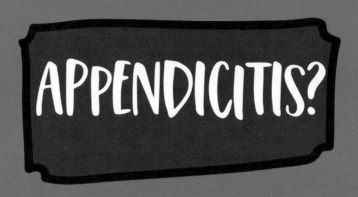

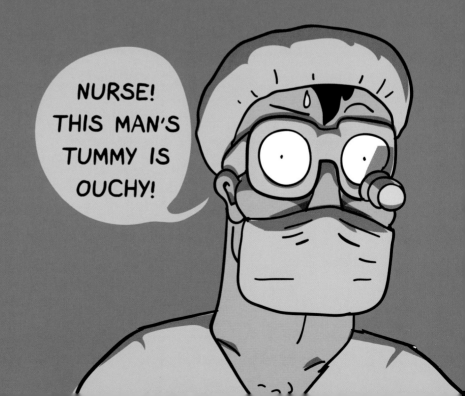

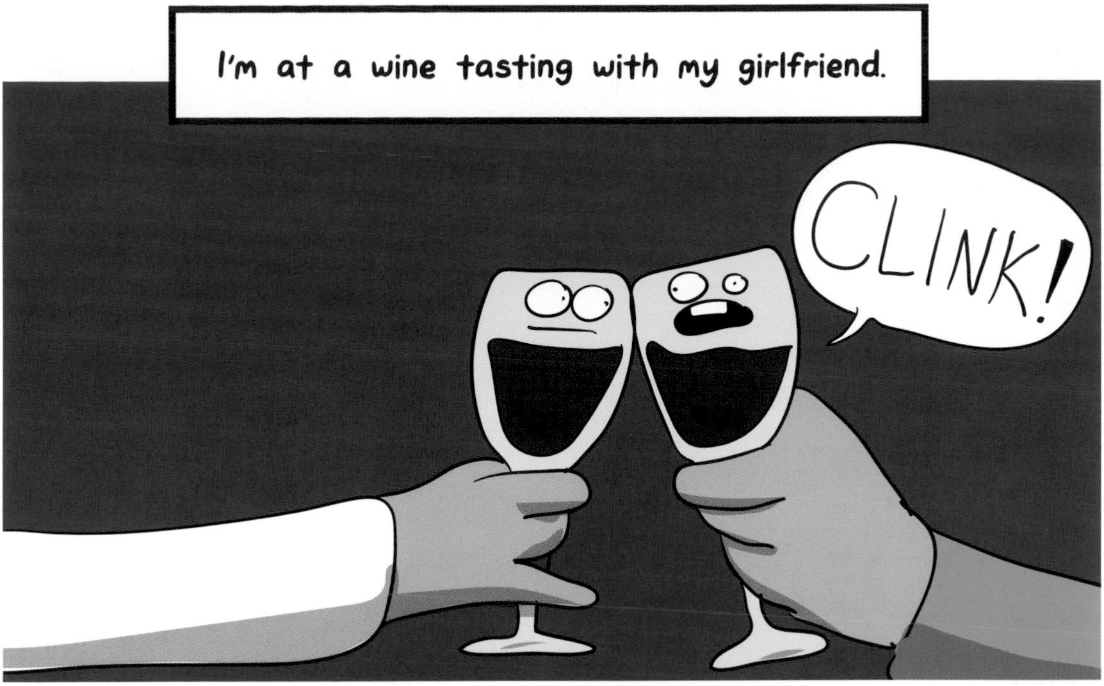
I'm at a wine tasting with my girlfriend.
CLINK!

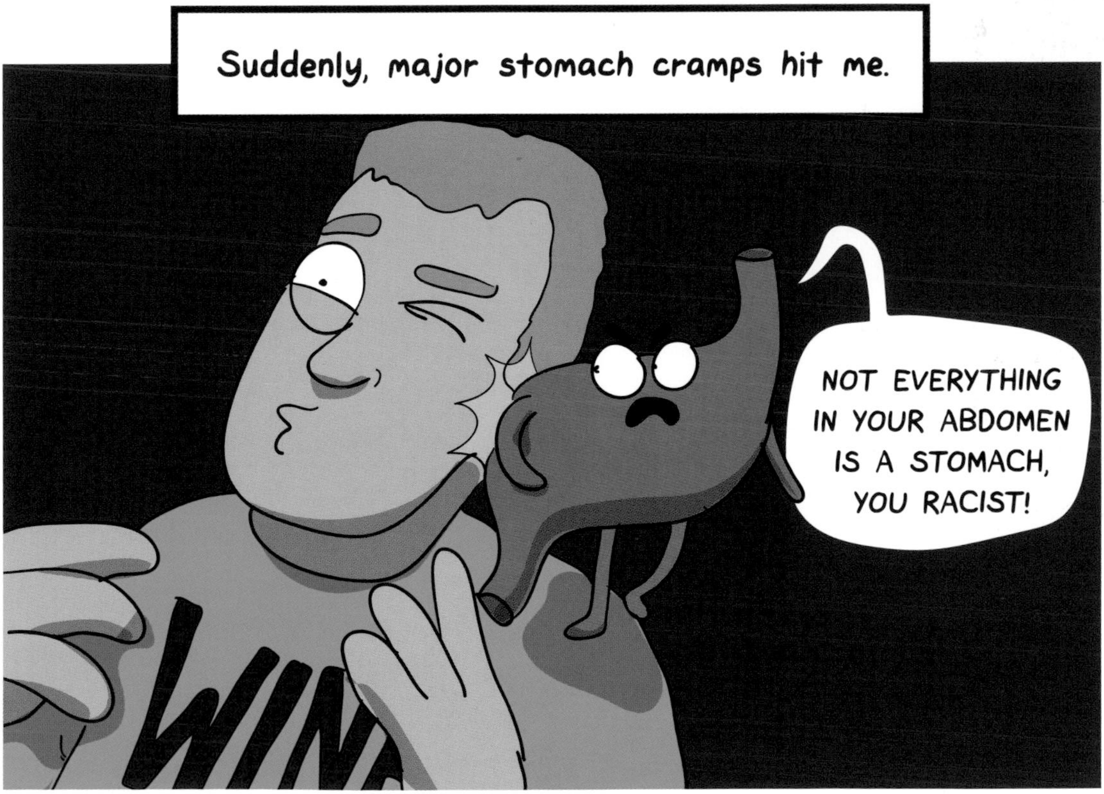
Suddenly, major stomach cramps hit me.
NOT EVERYTHING IN YOUR ABDOMEN IS A STOMACH, YOU RACIST!

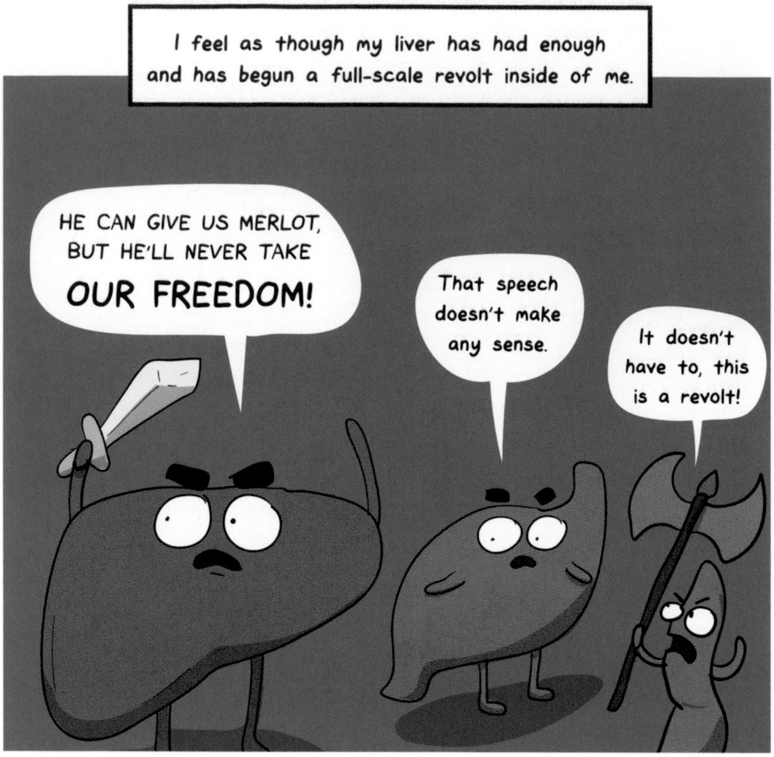
I feel as though my liver has had enough and has begun a full-scale revolt inside of me.
HE CAN GIVE US MERLOT, BUT HE'LL NEVER TAKE OUR FREEDOM!
That speech doesn't make any sense.
It doesn't have to, this is a revolt!

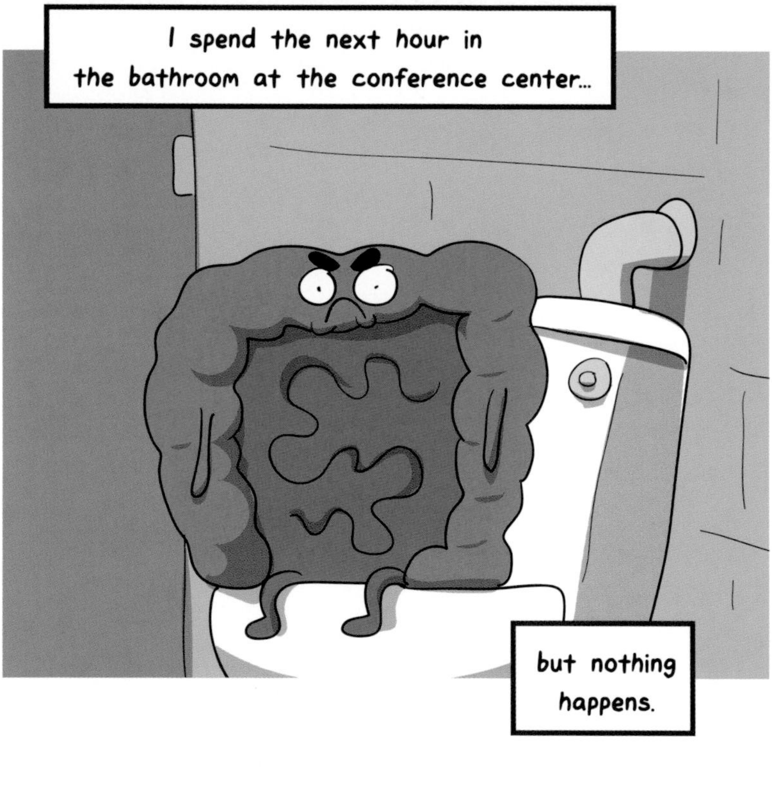
I spend the next hour in the bathroom at the conference center...
but nothing happens.

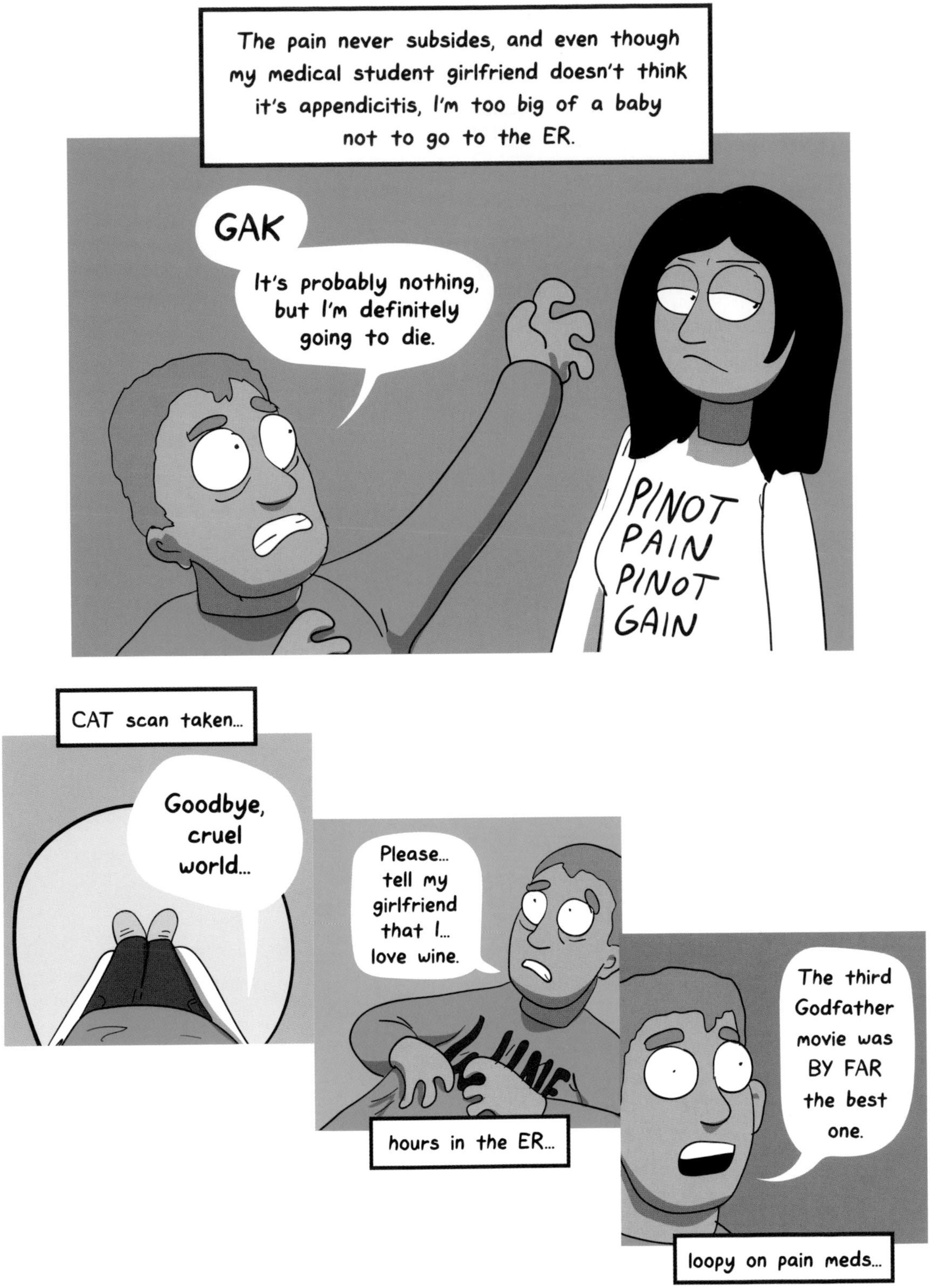
The pain never subsides, and even though my medical student girlfriend doesn't think it's appendicitis, I'm too big of a baby not to go to the ER.
GAK
It's probably nothing, but I'm definitely going to die.
PINOT PAIN PINOT GAIN
CAT scan taken...
Goodbye, cruel world...
Please... tell my girlfriend that I... love wine.
hours in the ER...
The third Godfather movie was BY FAR the best one.
loopy on pain meds...

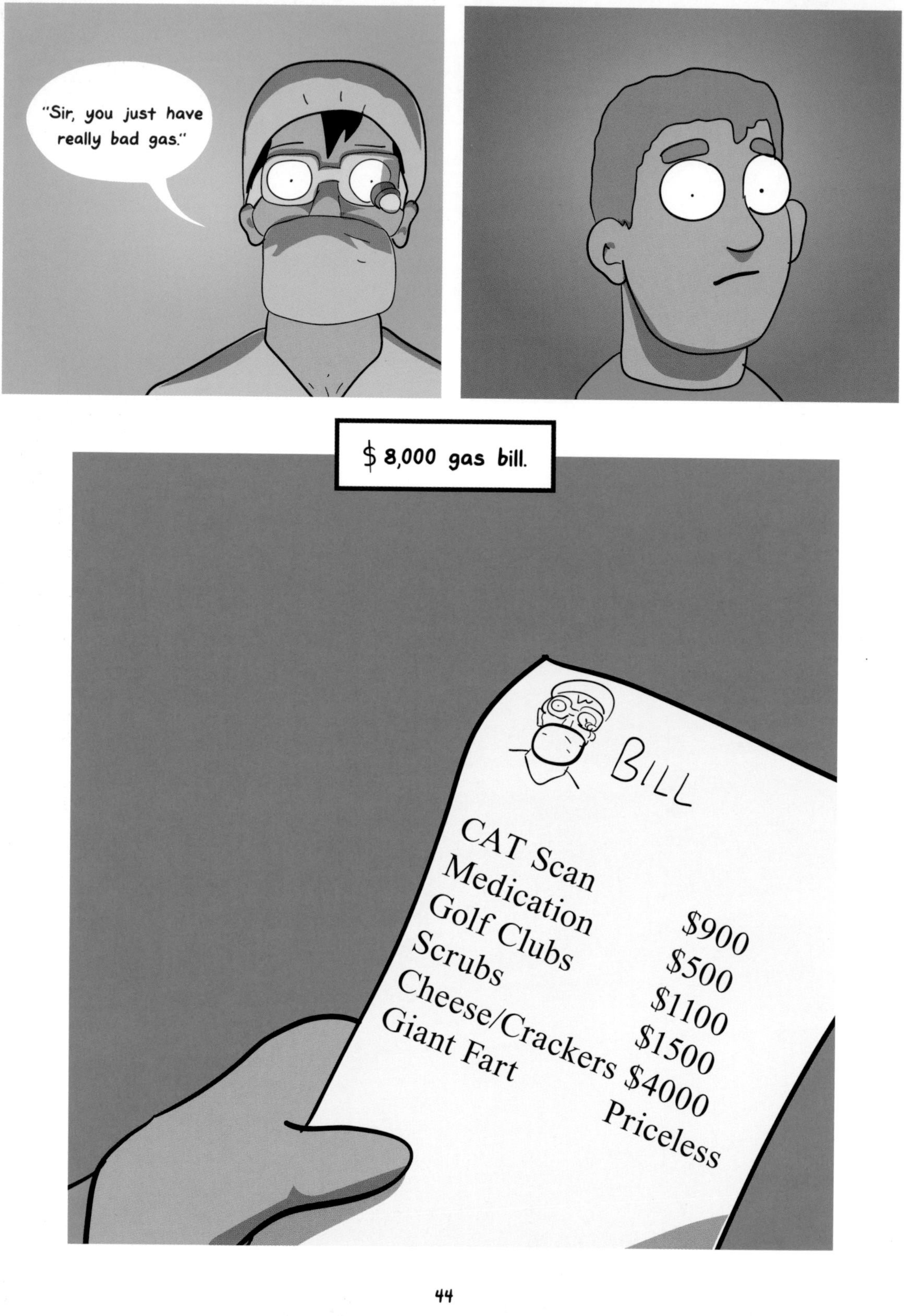
"Sir, you just have really bad gas."
$ 8,000 gas bill.
BILL
CAT Scan
Medication
Golf Clubs
Scrubs
Cheese/Crackers
Giant Fart
$900
$500
$1100
$1500
$4000
Priceless

CHAPTER 7

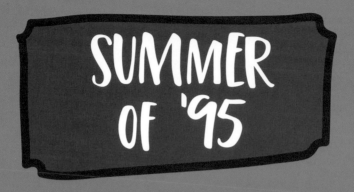

# SUMMER OF '95

told by Aine Maloney

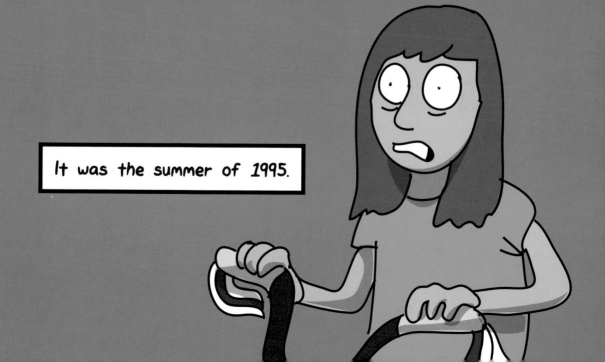

It was the summer of 1995.

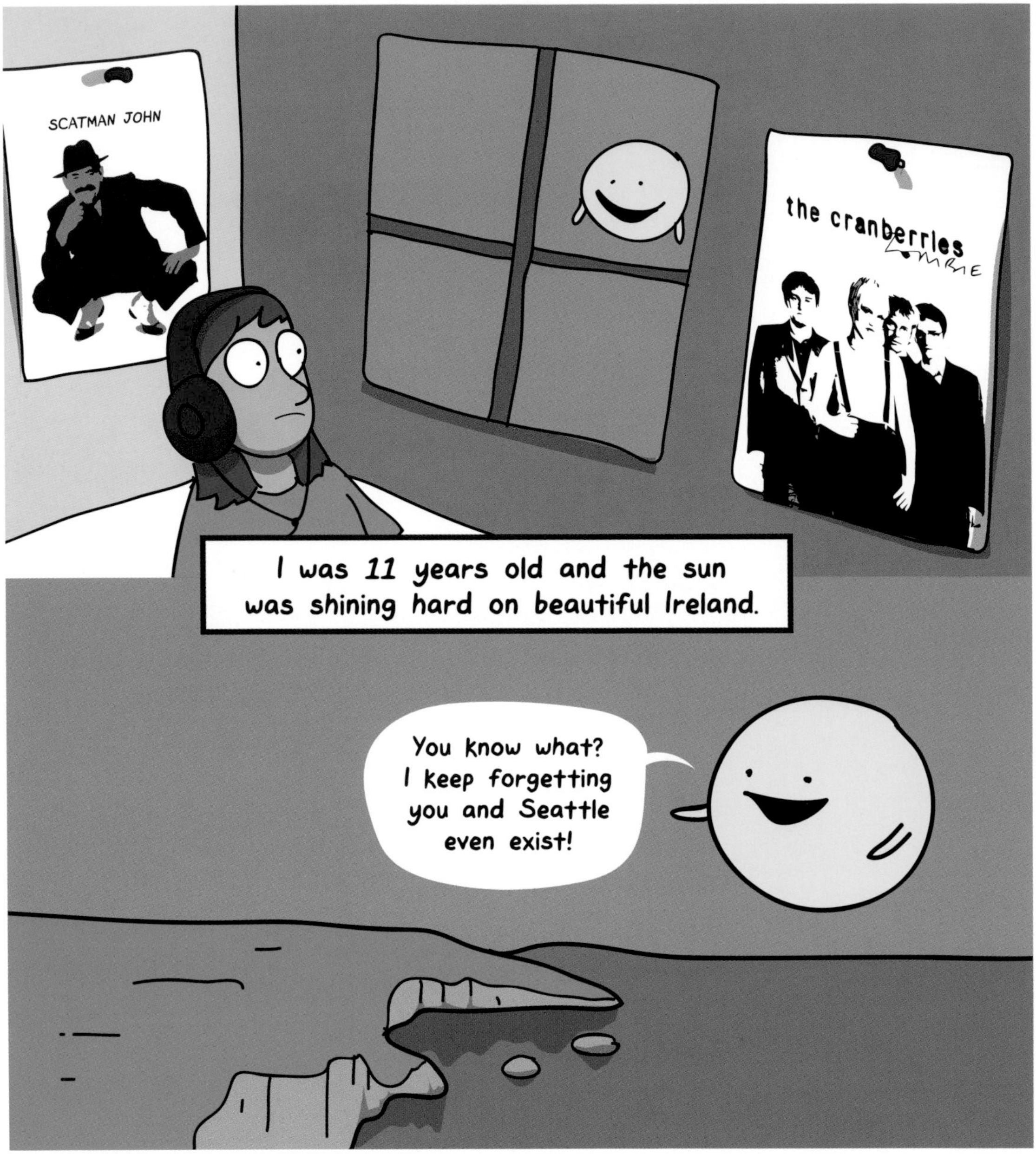
SCATMAN JOHN
the cranberries
ZOMBIE
I was 11 years old and the sun was shining hard on beautiful Ireland.
You know what? I keep forgetting you and Seattle even exist!

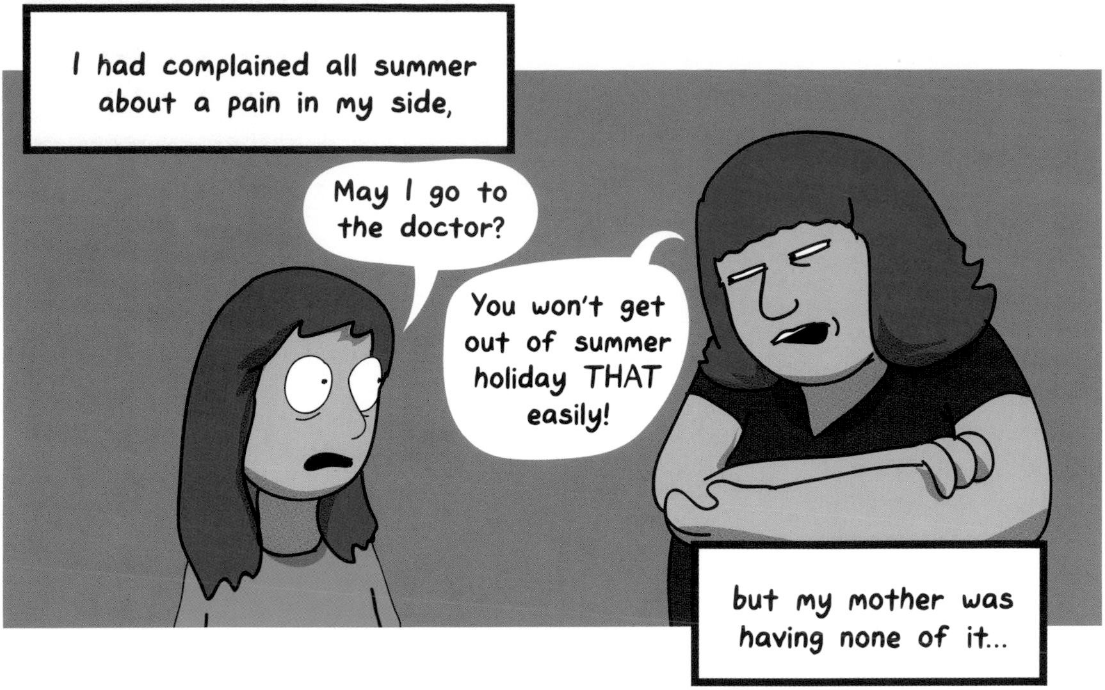
I had complained all summer about a pain in my side,
May I go to the doctor?
You won't get out of summer holiday THAT easily!
but my mother was having none of it...

The summer sun was there to be enjoyed, imaginary pains be damned!

I was made to cycle and swim and basically "enjoy" all that the summer had to offer... all the while coping with the ongoing pain in my right side...

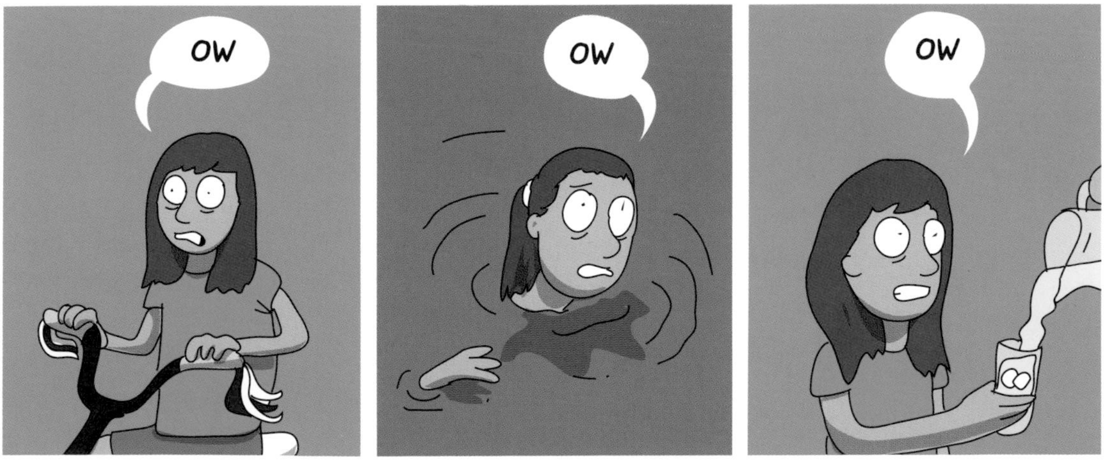
OW
OW
OW

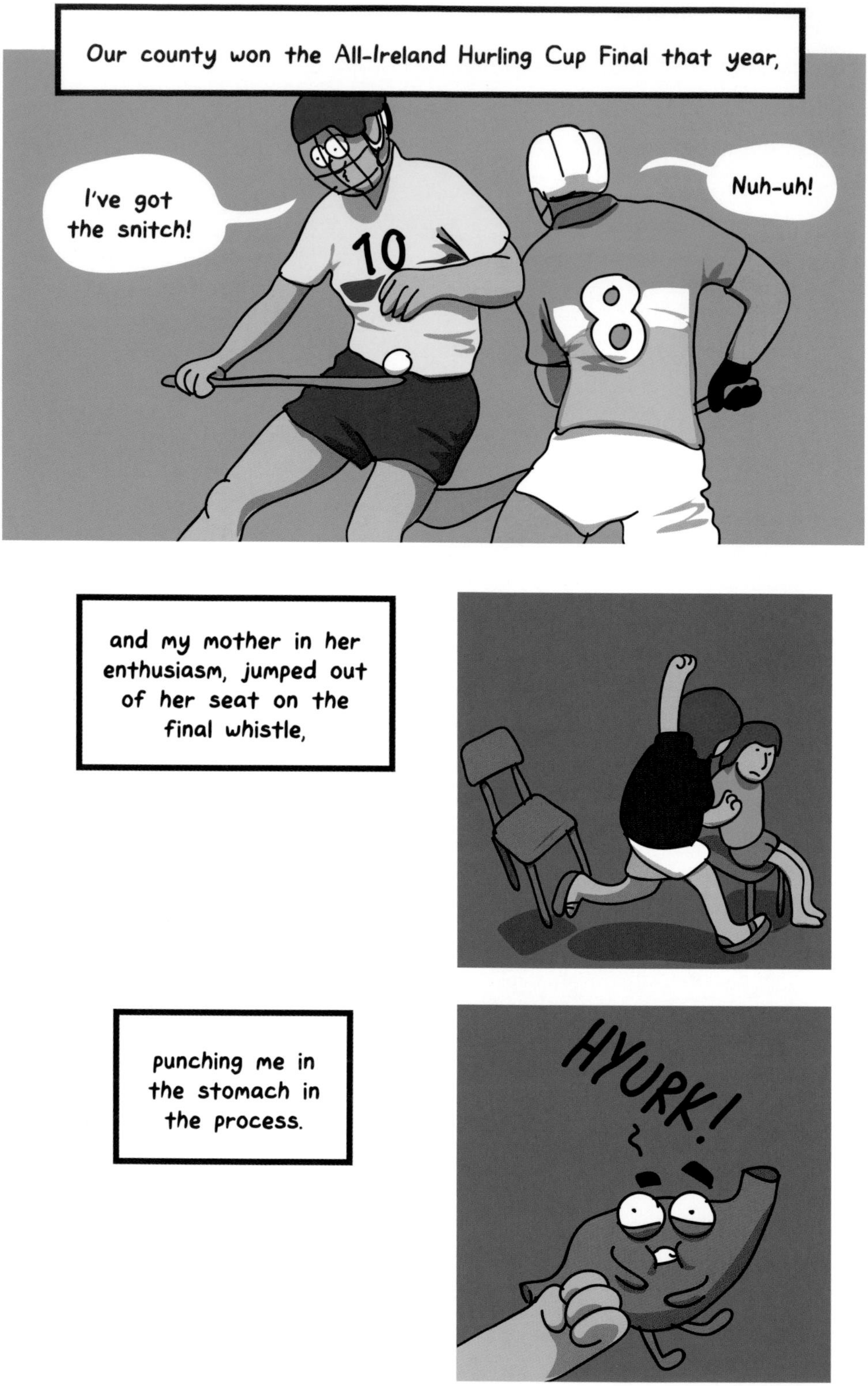
Our county won the All-Ireland Hurling Cup Final that year,
I've got the snitch!
Nuh-uh!
10
8
and my mother in her enthusiasm, jumped out of her seat on the final whistle,
punching me in the stomach in the process.
HYURK!

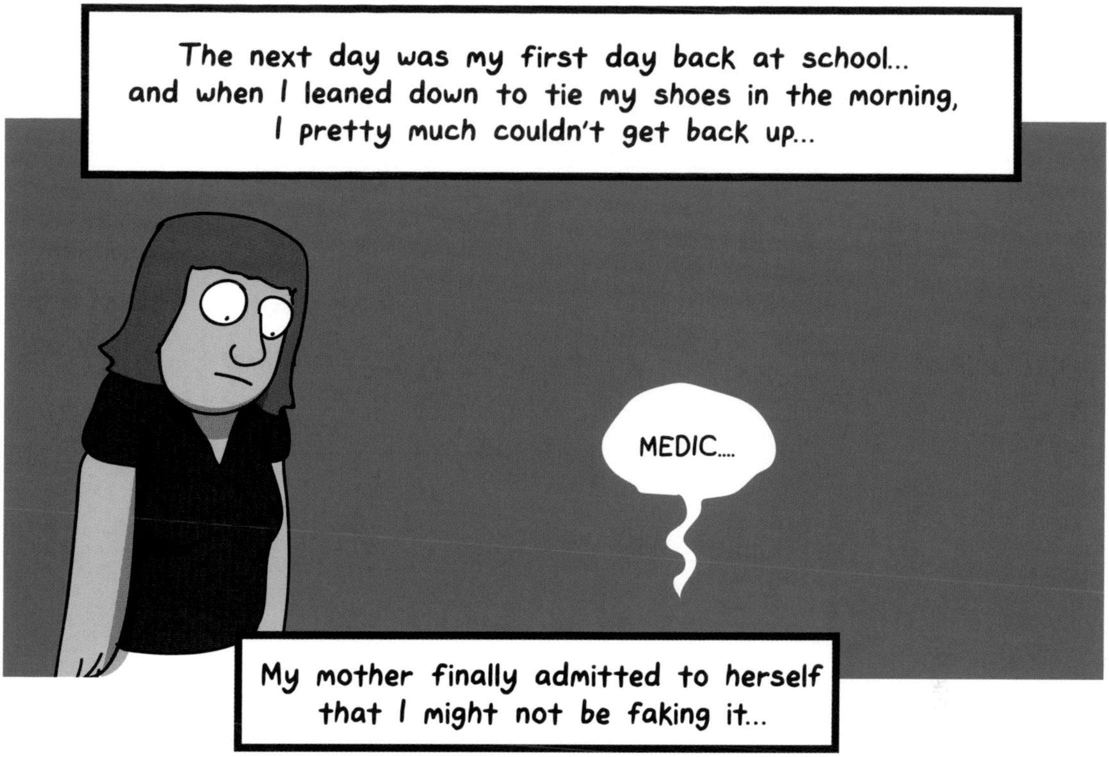
The next day was my first day back at school... and when I leaned down to tie my shoes in the morning, I pretty much couldn't get back up...
MEDIC....
My mother finally admitted to herself that I might not be faking it...

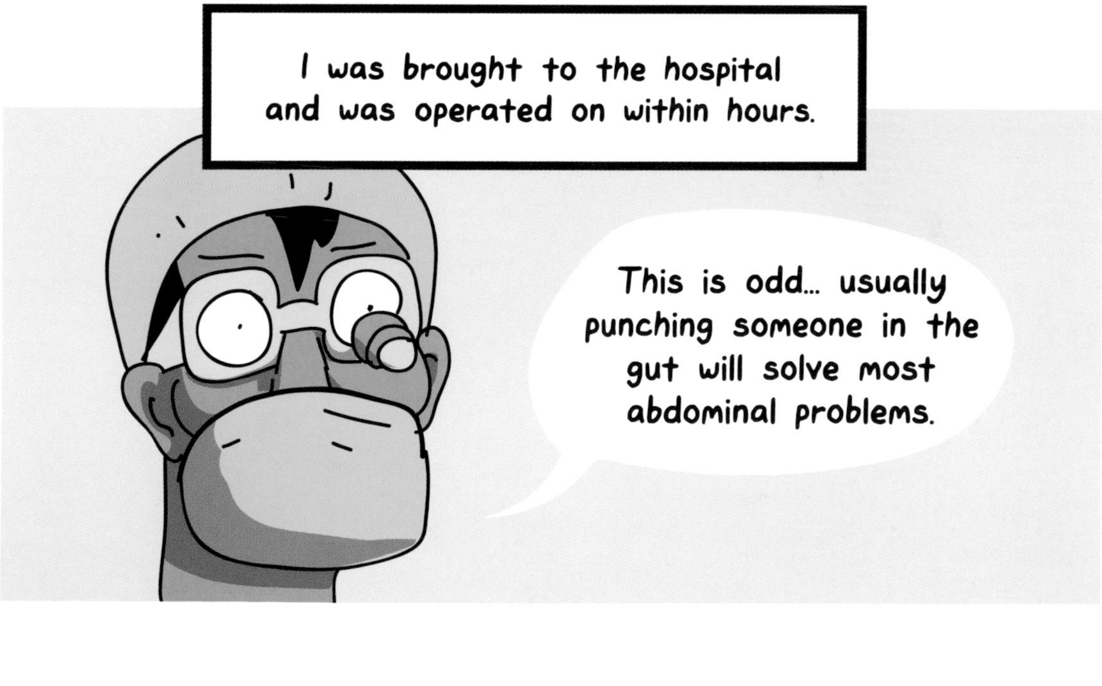
I was brought to the hospital and was operated on within hours.
This is odd... usually punching someone in the gut will solve most abdominal problems.

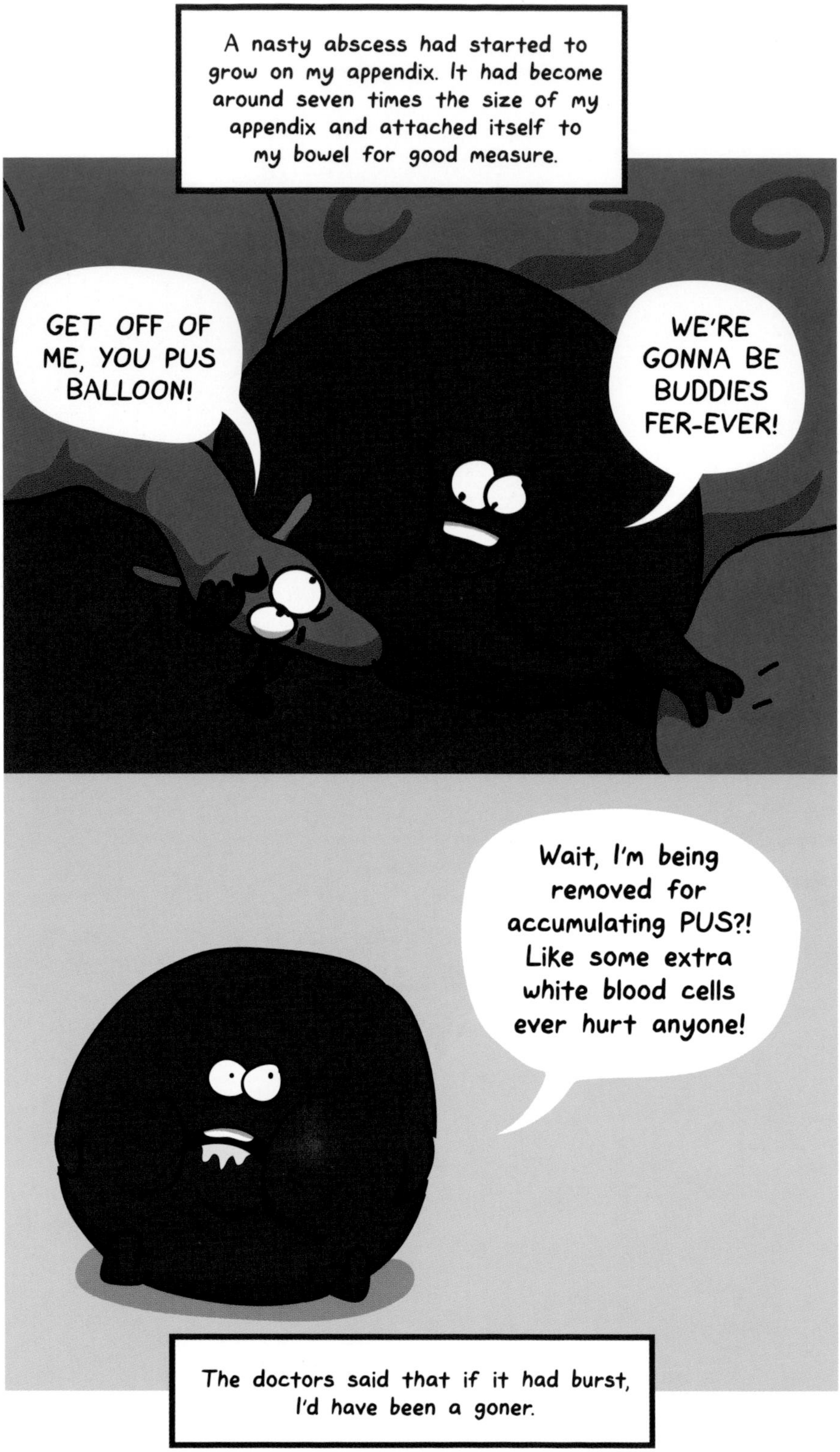
A nasty abscess had started to grow on my appendix. It had become around seven times the size of my appendix and attached itself to my bowel for good measure.
GET OFF OF ME, YOU PUS BALLOON!
WE'RE GONNA BE BUDDIES FER-EVER!
Wait, I'm being removed for accumulating PUS?! Like some extra white blood cells ever hurt anyone!
The doctors said that if it had burst, I'd have been a goner.

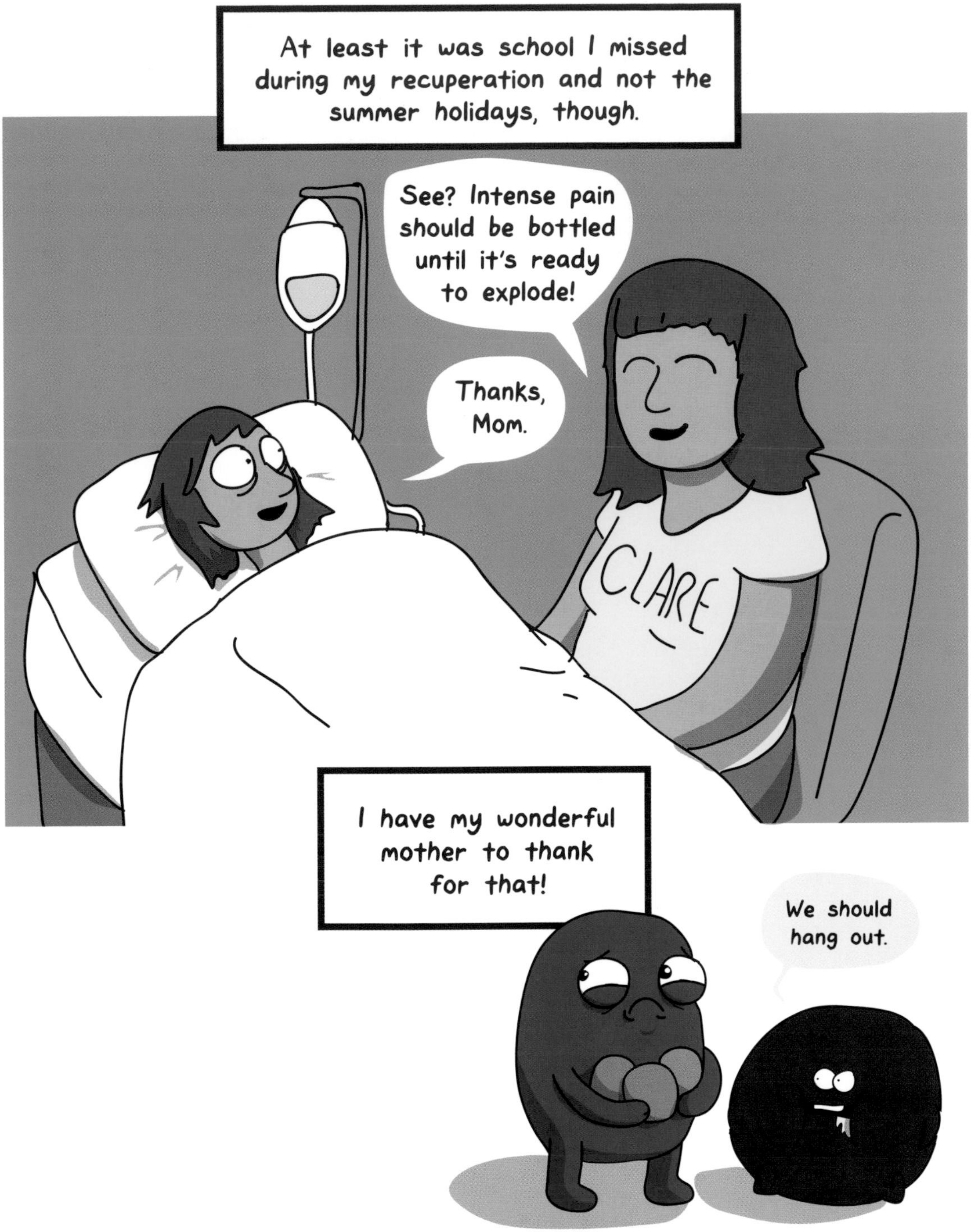

At least it was school I missed during my recuperation and not the summer holidays, though.
See? Intense pain should be bottled until it's ready to explode!
Thanks, Mom.
CLARE
I have my wonderful mother to thank for that!
We should hang out.

# CHAPTER 8

# THE GEOLOGIST

told by Laura Bax

For many years, I had been suffering increasing pain in my lower right back.

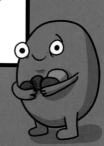

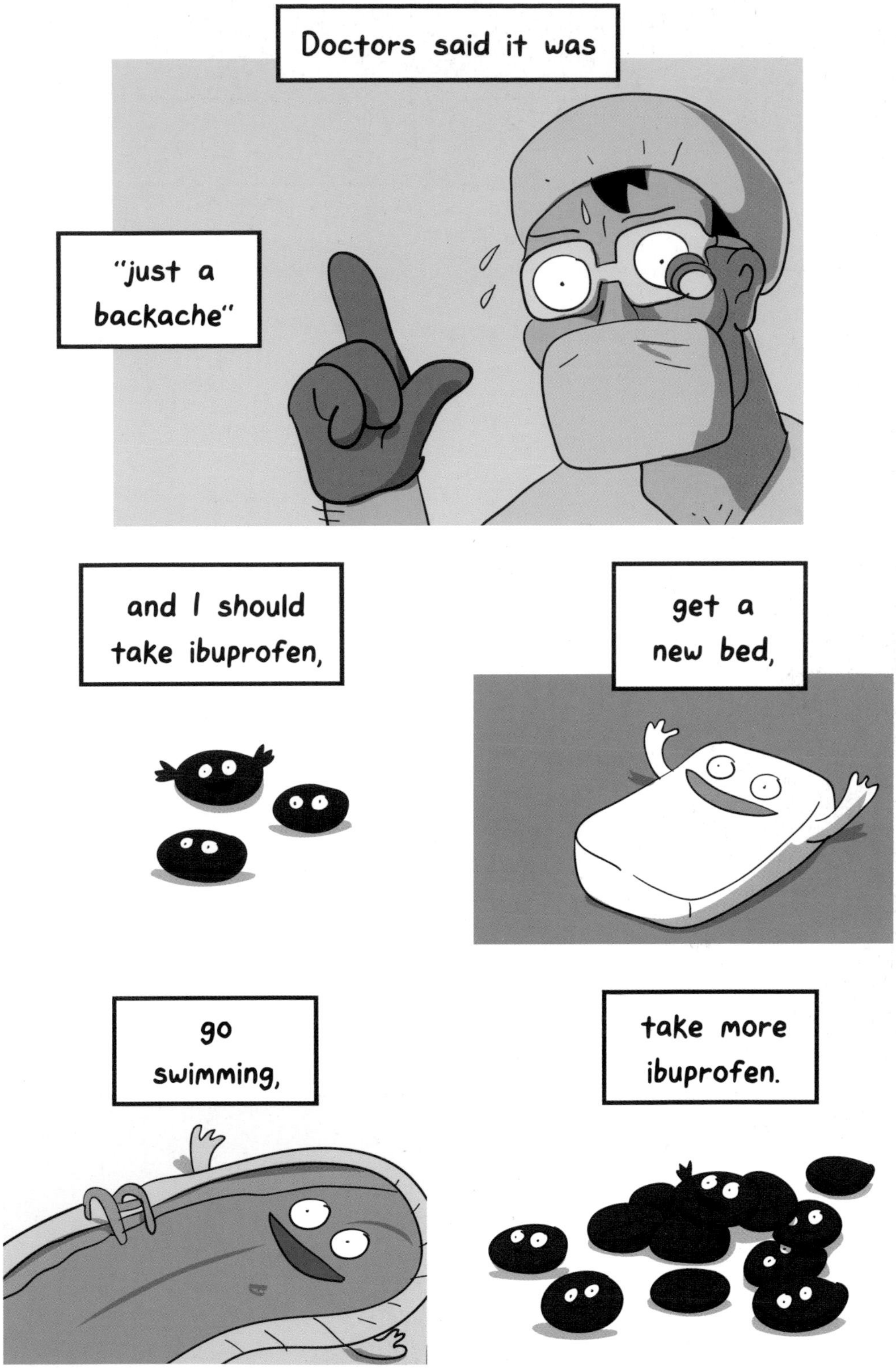
Doctors said it was
"just a backache"
and I should take ibuprofen,
get a new bed,
go swimming,
take more ibuprofen.

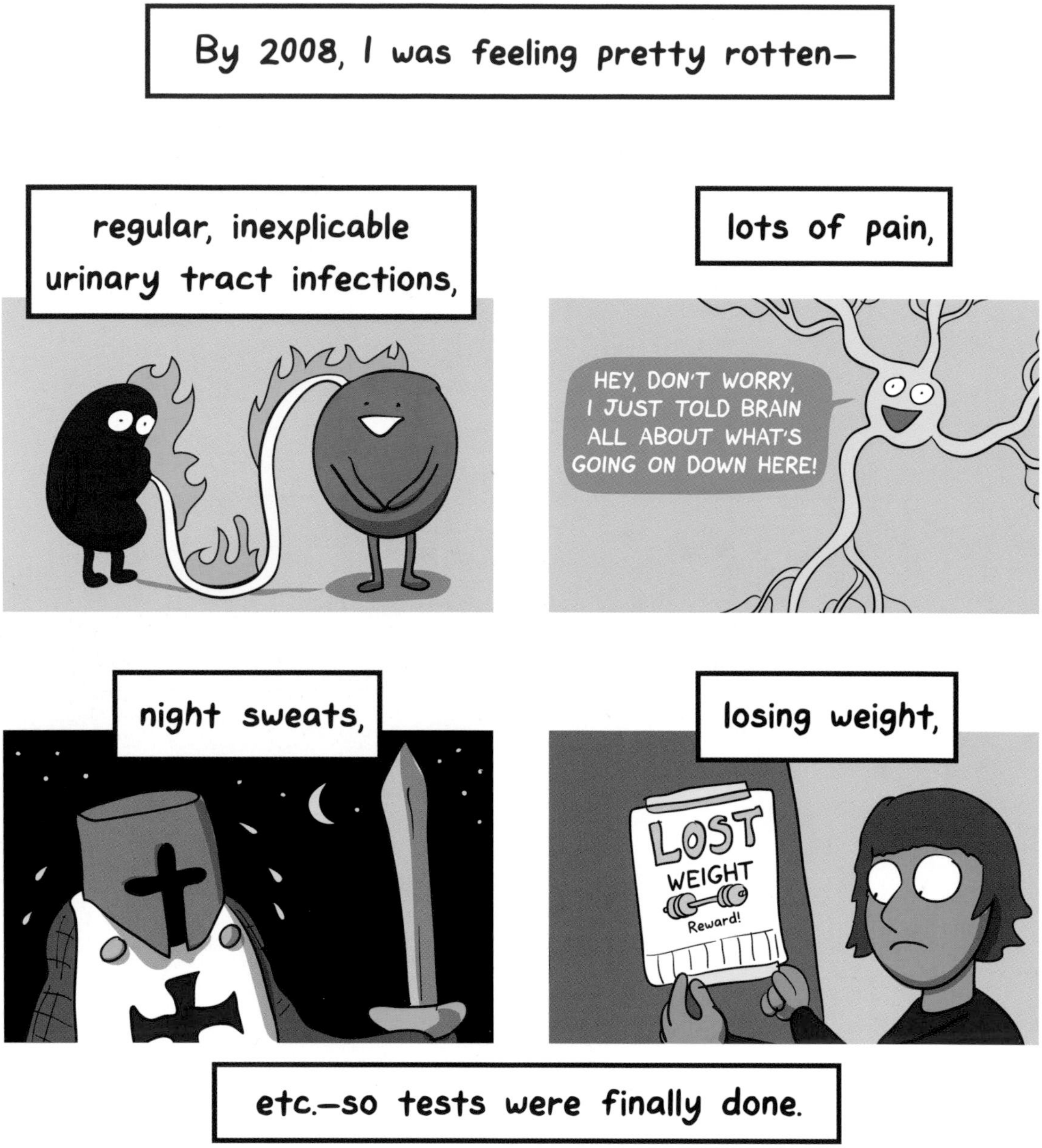
By 2008, I was feeling pretty rotten—
regular, inexplicable urinary tract infections,
lots of pain,
HEY, DON'T WORRY, I JUST TOLD BRAIN ALL ABOUT WHAT'S GOING ON DOWN HERE!
night sweats,
losing weight,
LOST WEIGHT
Reward!
etc.—so tests were finally done.

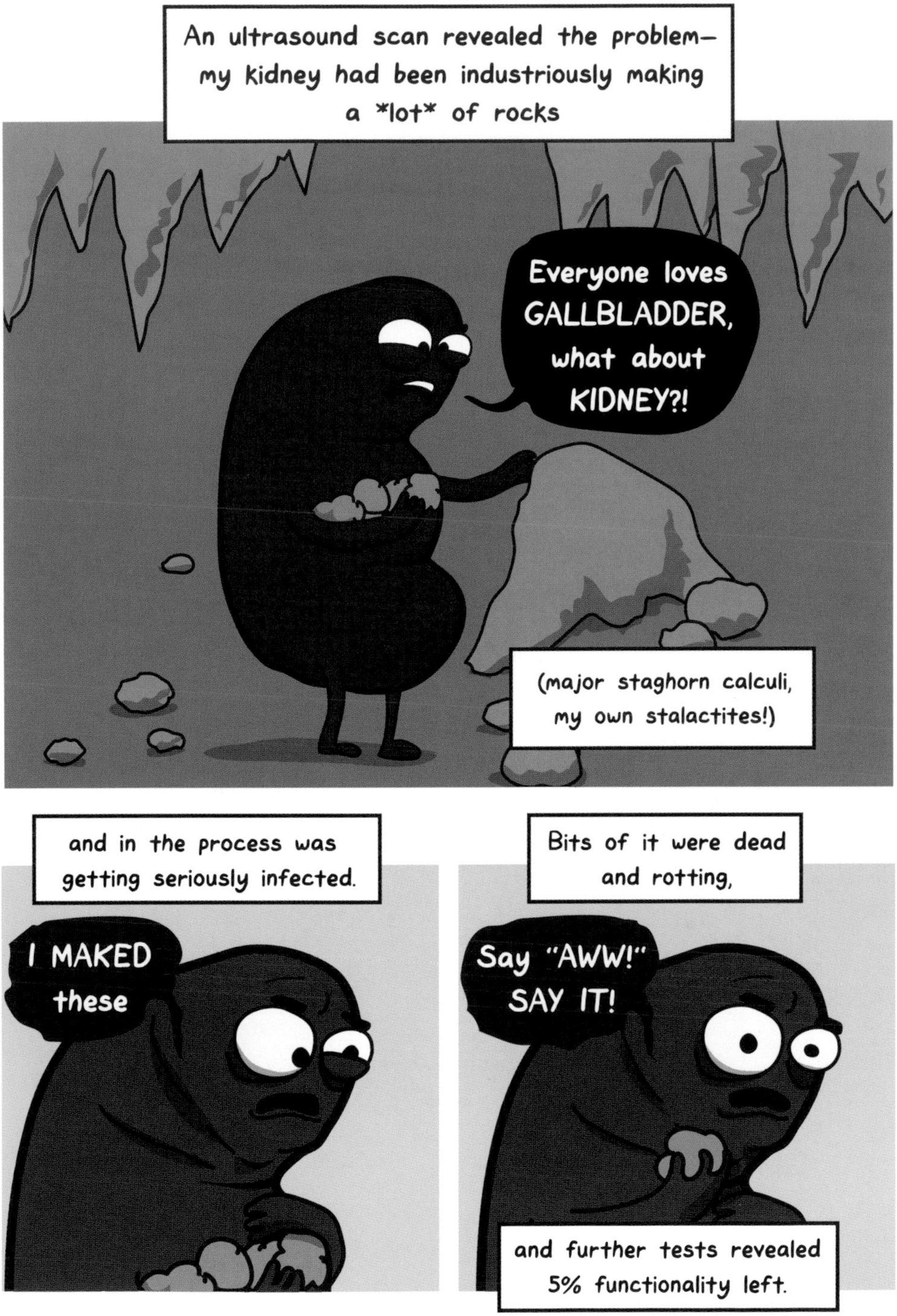
An ultrasound scan revealed the problem—
my kidney had been industriously making
a *lot* of rocks
Everyone loves GALLBLADDER, what about KIDNEY?!
(major staghorn calculi, my own stalactites!)
and in the process was getting seriously infected.
I MAKED these
Bits of it were dead and rotting,
Say "AWW!" SAY IT!
and further tests revealed 5% functionality left.

I had to have my right kidney completely removed in June 2009, after many tests and waiting lists. The consultant said he'd never seen anything like it, and it could have burst and killed me at any time over the last couple years.

Medical students were sent to study me, and the doctor who performed the original ultrasound fetched her boss to see it because it was so weird.

I concur with the weirdness!

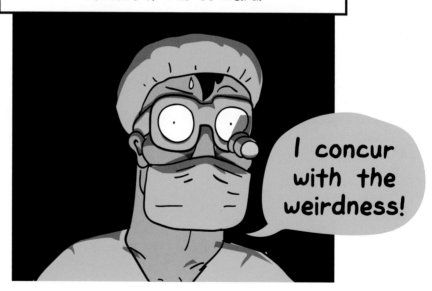

## Epilogue

The following year (2010), after recovery from all that, the pain returned to my *left* side and I ended up in the hospital again—

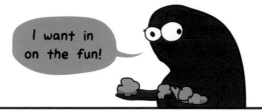

I want in on the fun!

the "day surgery" to remove the new pebbles in my left kidney went horribly wrong, leaving me with visceral scarring, which hurts to this day.

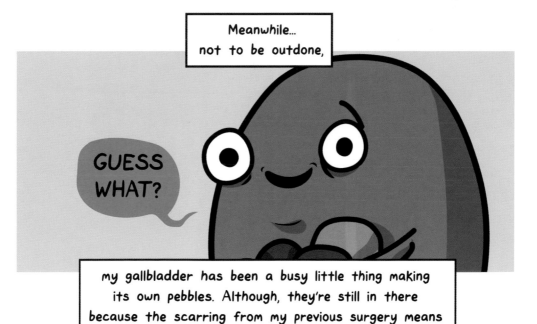

Meanwhile... not to be outdone,

GUESS WHAT?

my gallbladder has been a busy little thing making its own pebbles. Although, they're still in there because the scarring from my previous surgery means that the removal can't be done by keyhole,

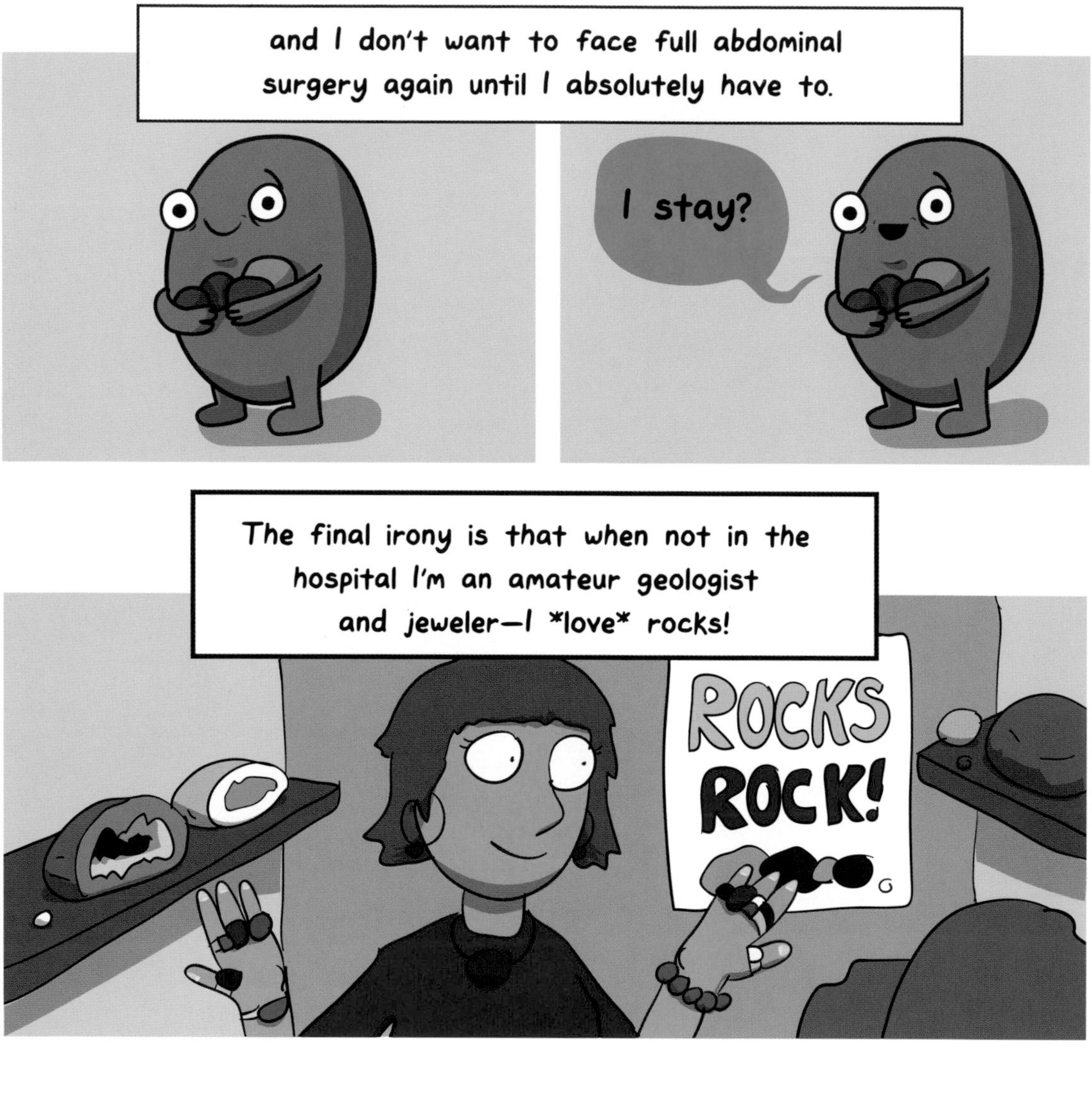
and I don't want to face full abdominal surgery again until I absolutely have to.
I stay?
The final irony is that when not in the hospital I'm an amateur geologist and jeweler—I *love* rocks!
ROCKS ROCK!

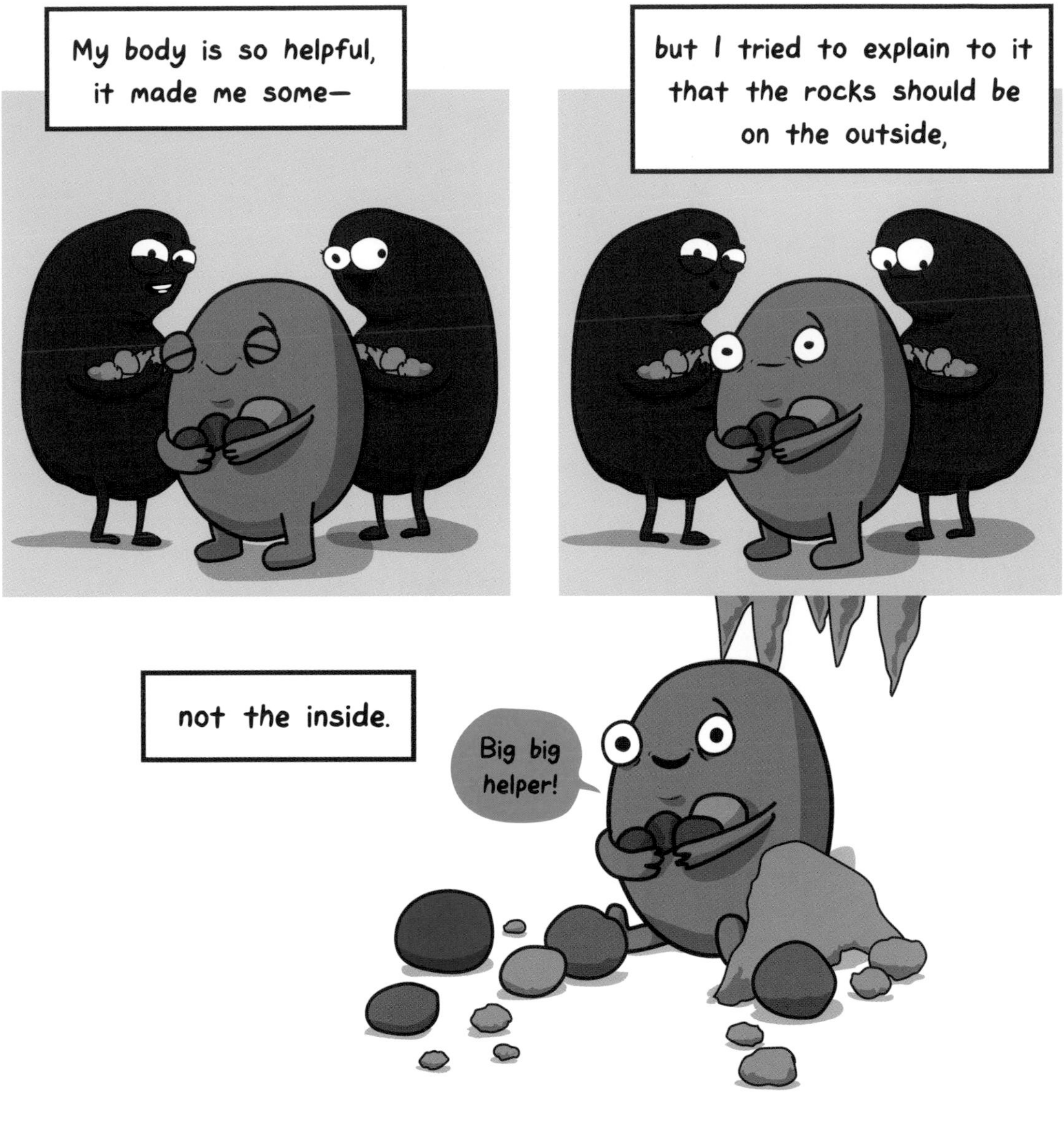
My body is so helpful, it made me some—
but I tried to explain to it that the rocks should be on the outside,
not the inside.
Big big helper!

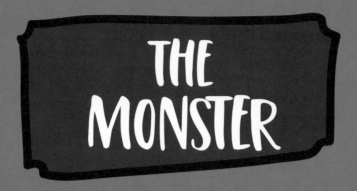

# CHAPTER 9

# THE MONSTER

## told by Casie Habetler

I was sitting in the waiting room of a children's hospital, dressed up and nervously holding my folder that contained my résumé and credentials for the job I was about to interview for.

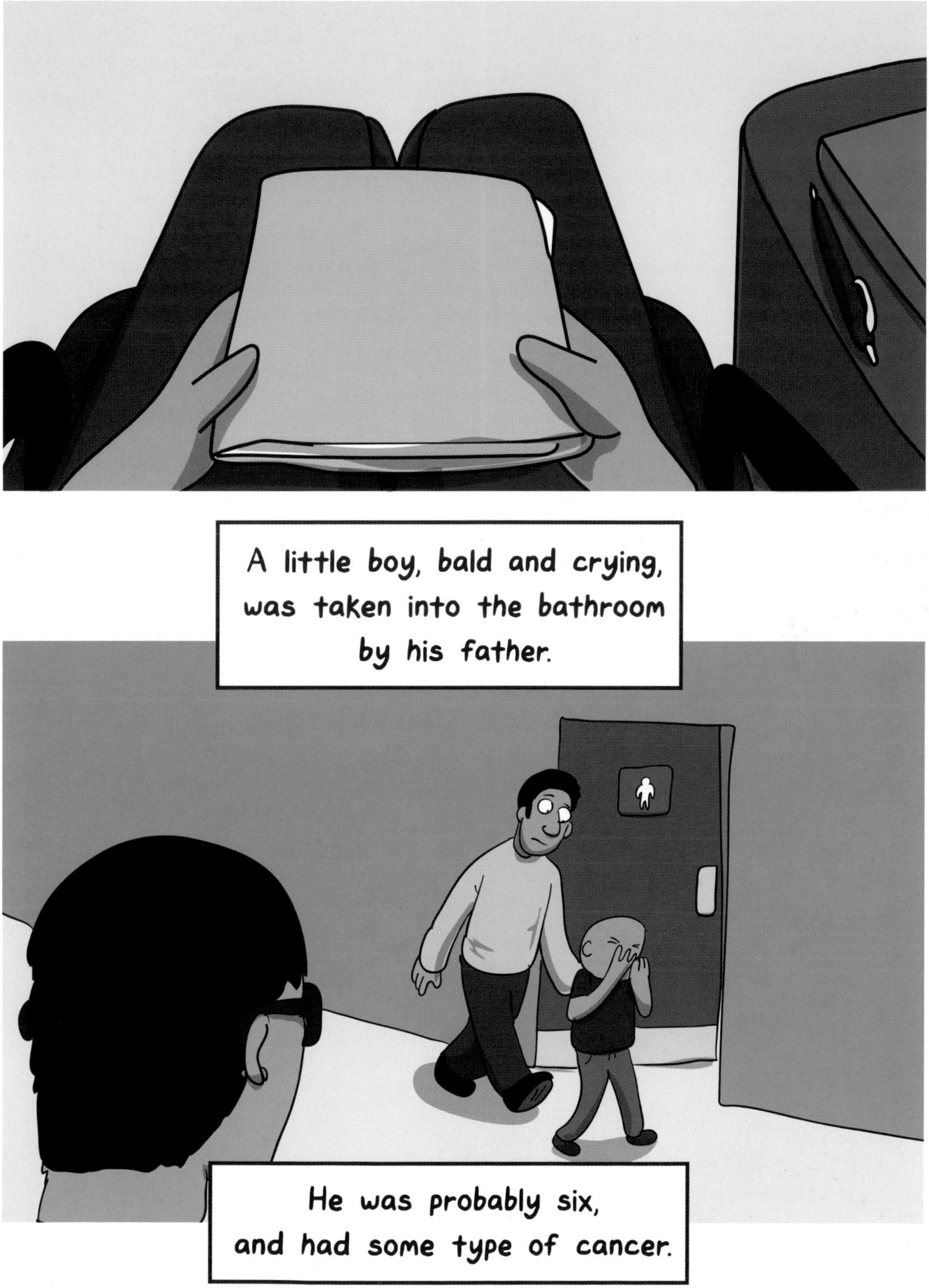
A little boy, bald and crying, was taken into the bathroom by his father.
He was probably six, and had some type of cancer.

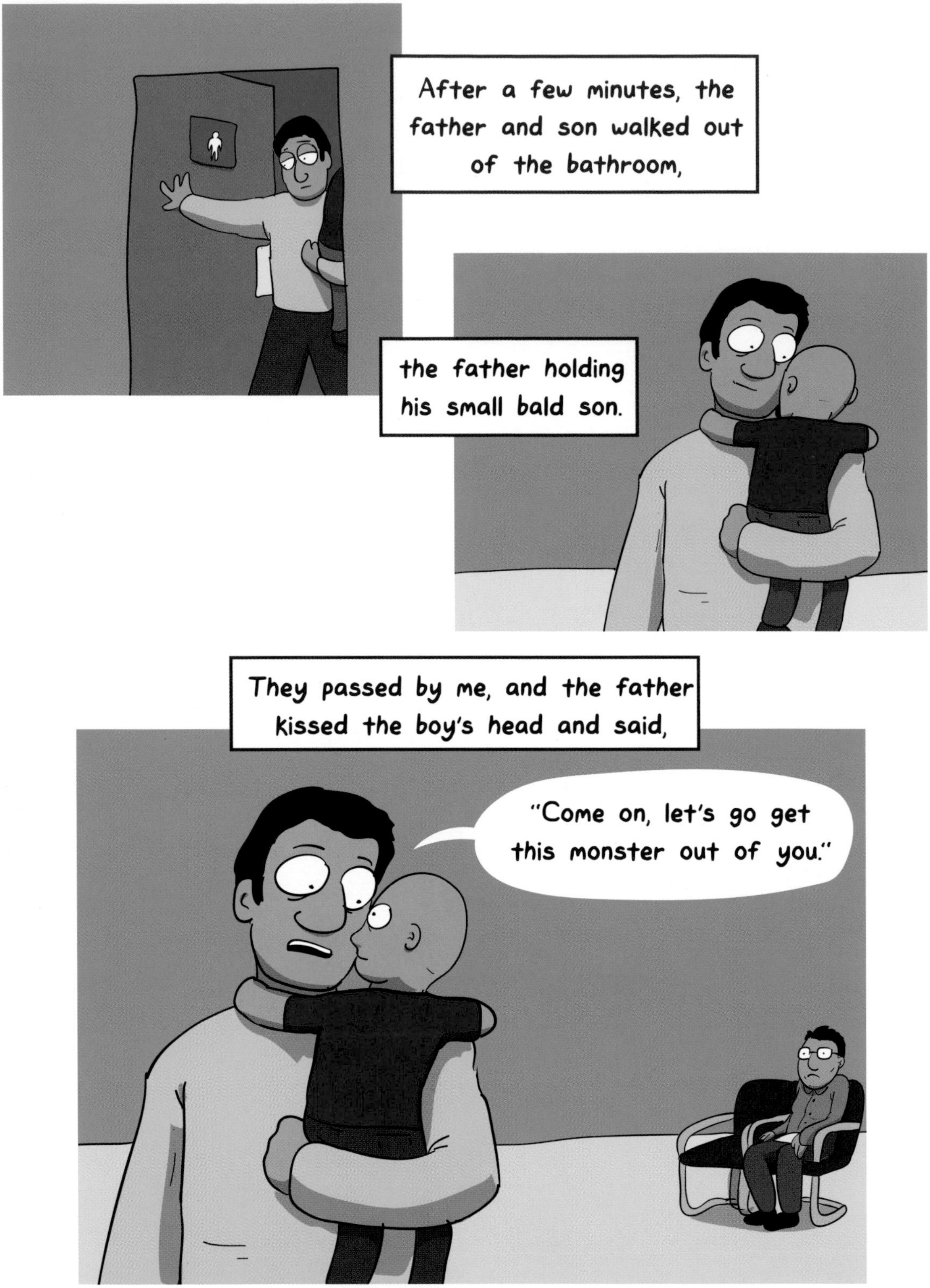
After a few minutes, the father and son walked out of the bathroom,
the father holding his small bald son.
They passed by me, and the father kissed the boy's head and said,
"Come on, let's go get this monster out of you."

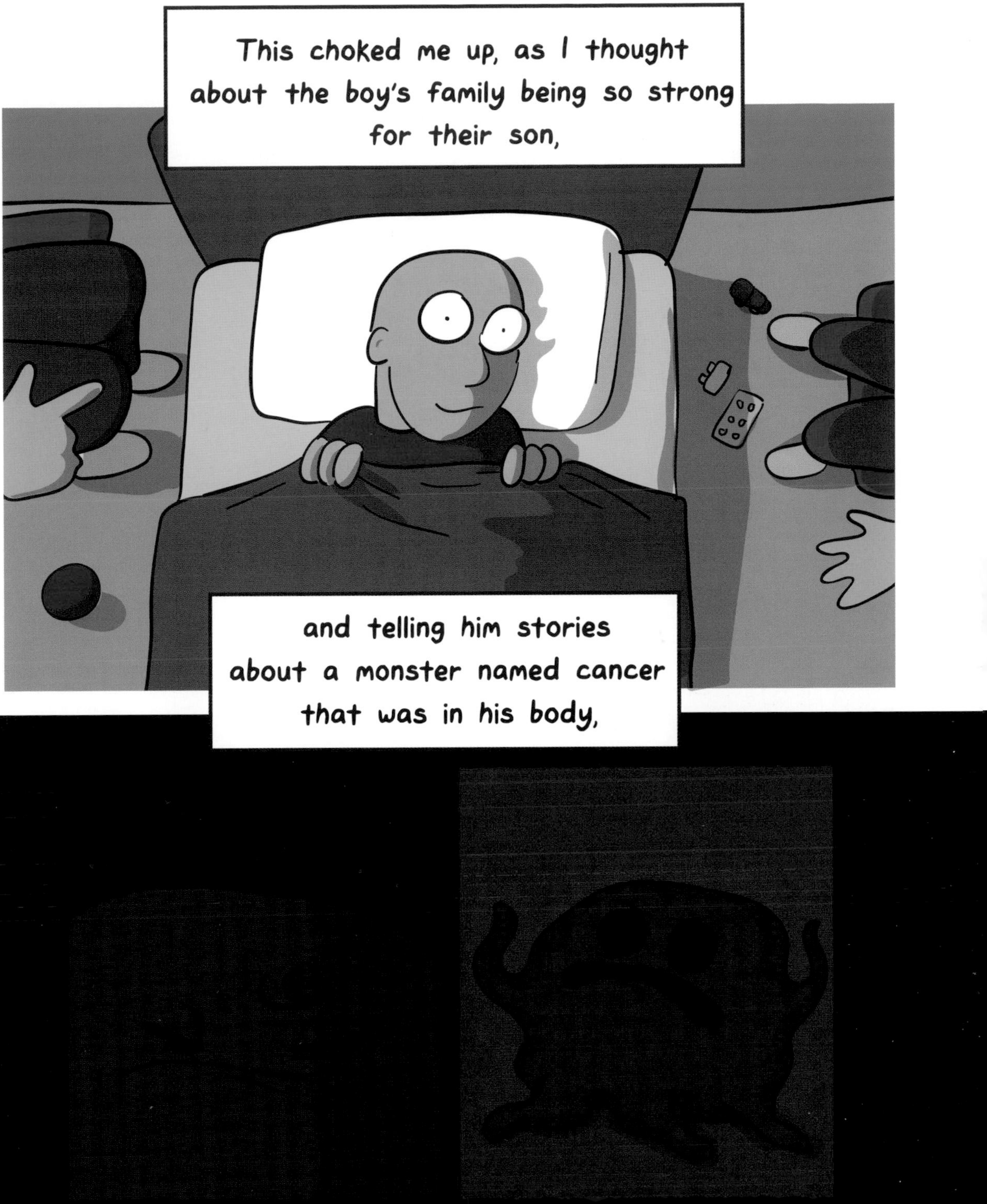
This choked me up, as I thought about the boy's family being so strong for their son,
and telling him stories about a monster named cancer that was in his body,

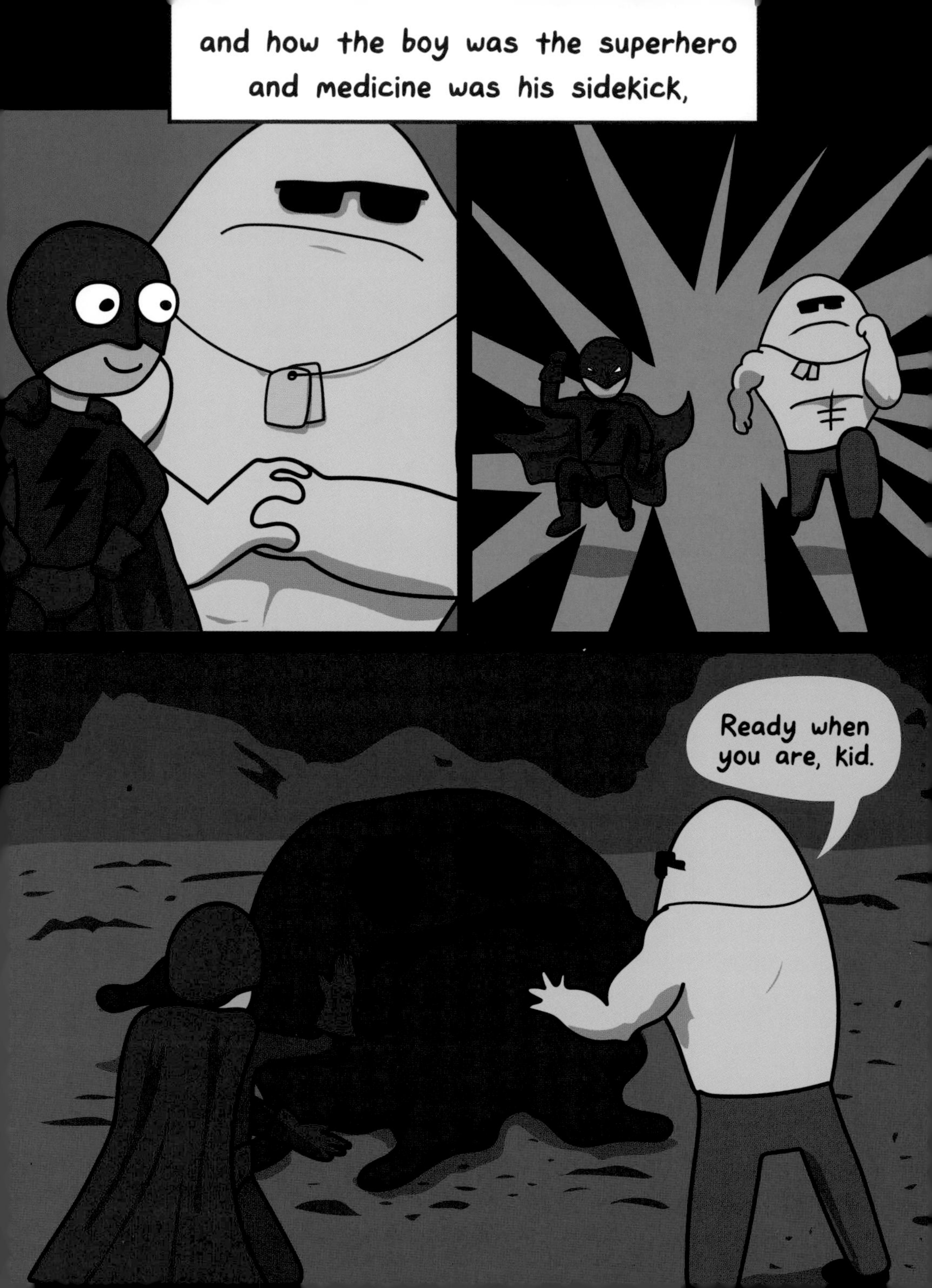
and how the boy was the superhero
and medicine was his sidekick,
Ready when you are, kid.

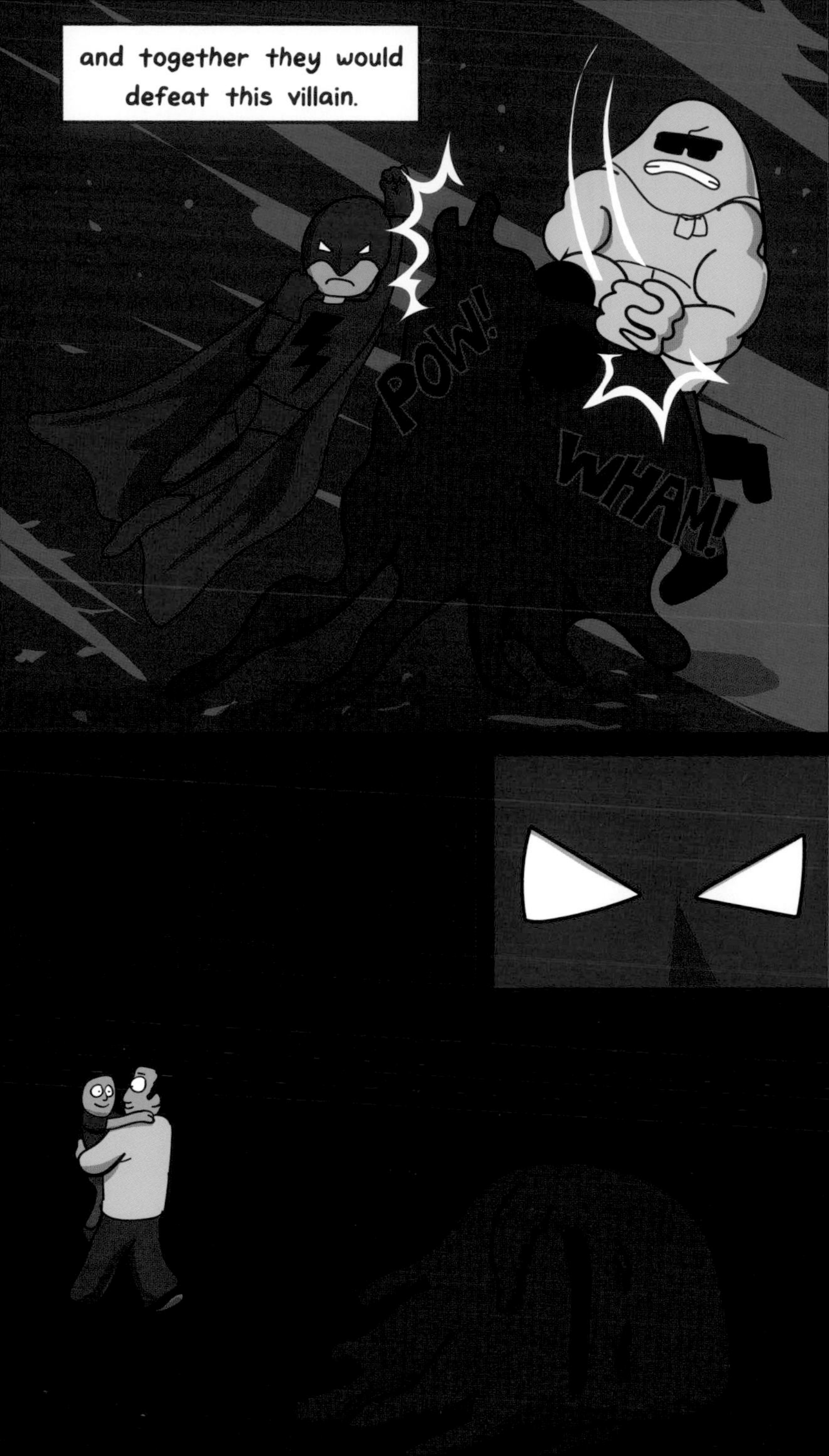
and together they would defeat this villain.
POW!
WHAM!

Although it's not much of a medical story, it's something that warms my heart and breaks it at the same time.

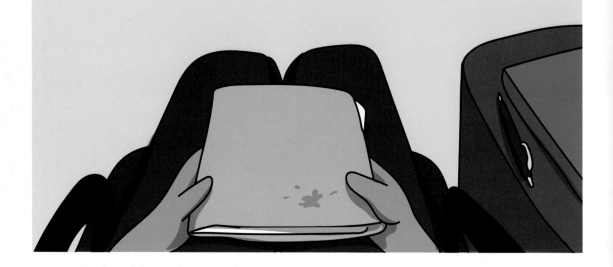

Seeing the parents of sick children being so strong and supportive is what inspires me to keep going in my medical career.

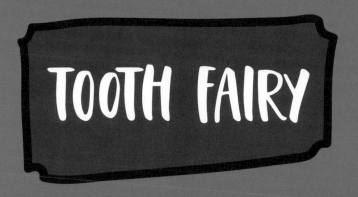

**told by Mad Doc D**

When my cousin was young,
she asked me why the tooth fairy
is interested in the teeth...

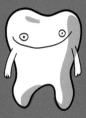

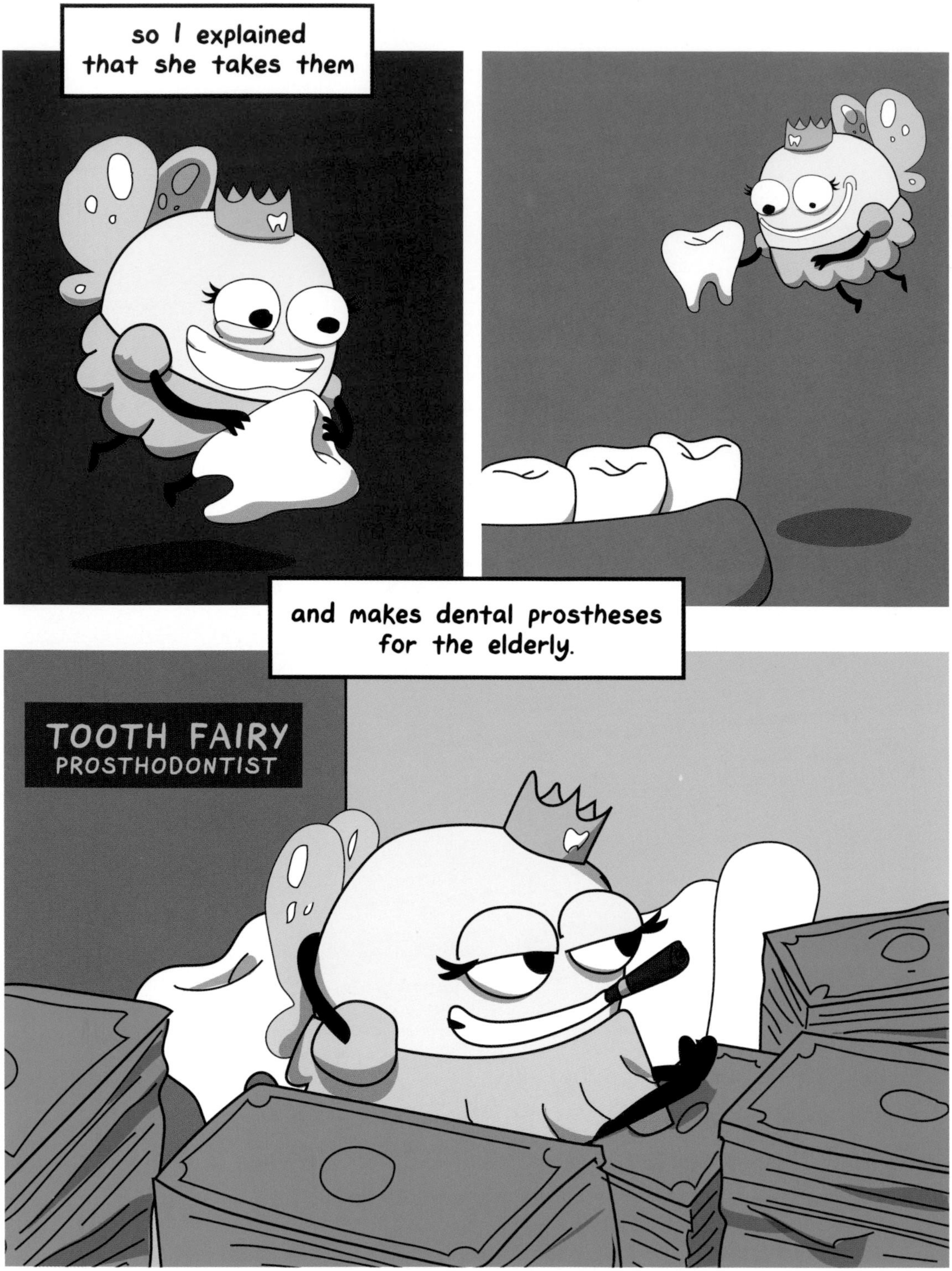
so I explained that she takes them
and makes dental prostheses for the elderly.
TOOTH FAIRY
PROSTHODONTIST

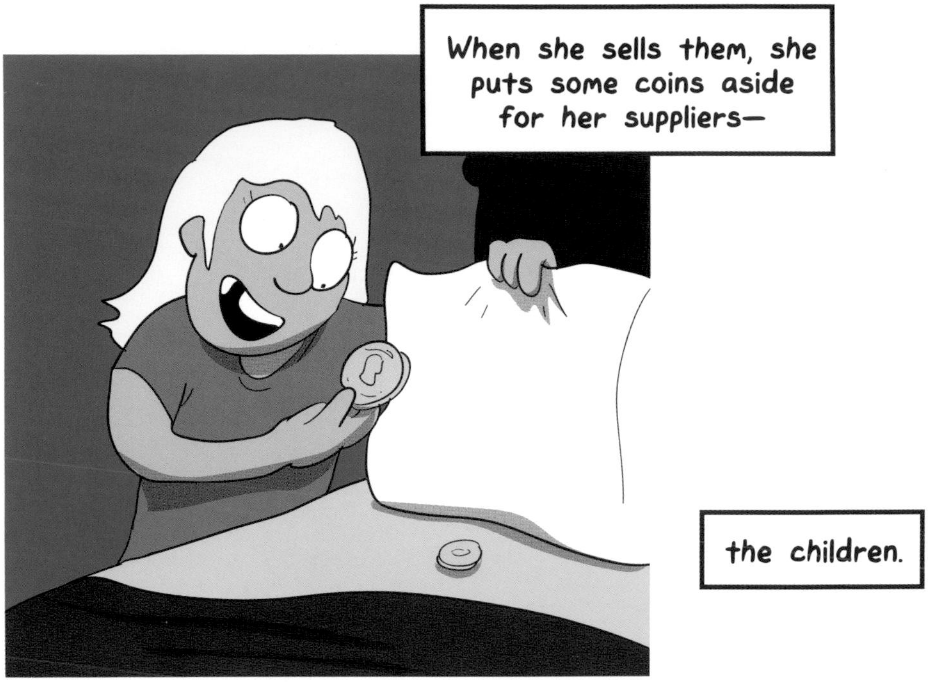
When she sells them, she puts some coins aside for her suppliers—
the children.

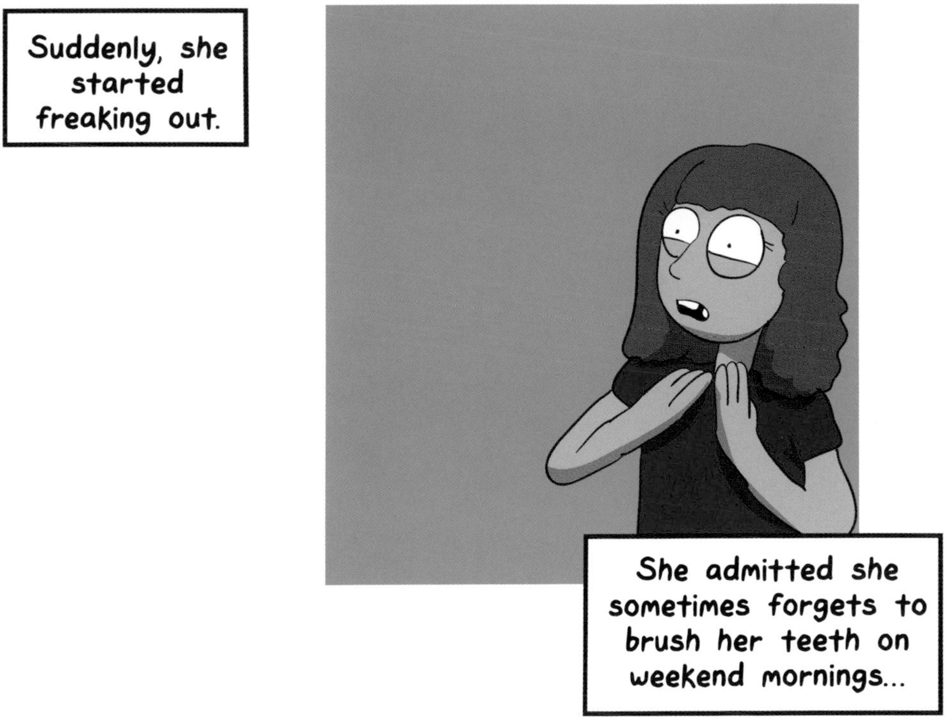
Suddenly, she started freaking out.
She admitted she sometimes forgets to brush her teeth on weekend mornings...

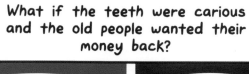

What if the teeth were carious and the old people wanted their money back?

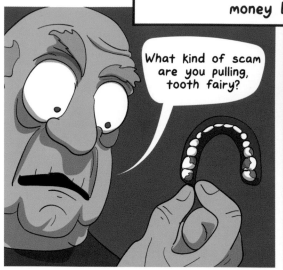

What kind of scam are you pulling, tooth fairy?

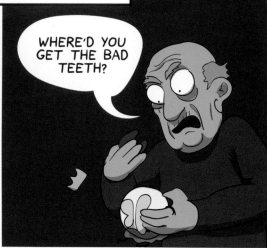

WHERE'D YOU GET THE BAD TEETH?

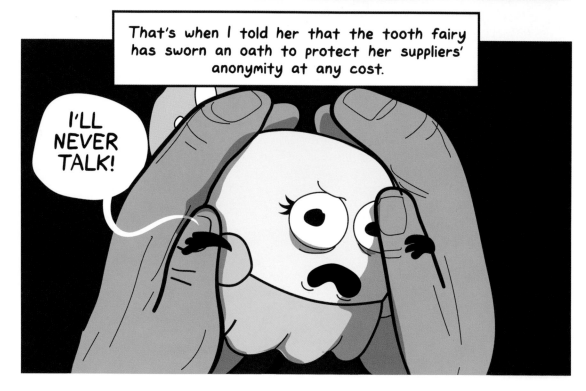

That's when I told her that the tooth fairy has sworn an oath to protect her suppliers' anonymity at any cost.

I'LL NEVER TALK!

For quite some time,
she would stare at
old people on the streets,

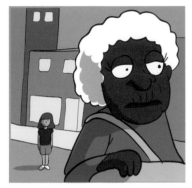

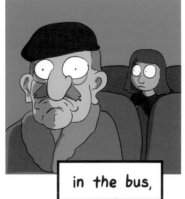

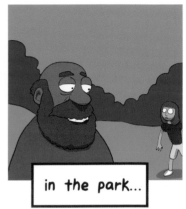

in the bus,

in the park...

trying to get a glimpse
at their teeth,

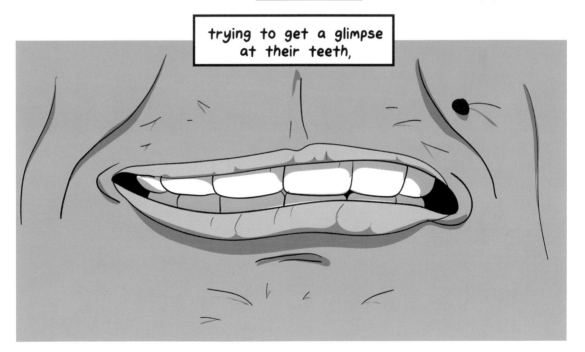

to see if there was
one of hers among them.

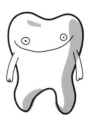

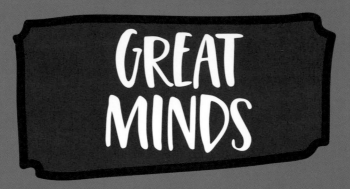

# CHAPTER 11

# GREAT MINDS

## told by Joel

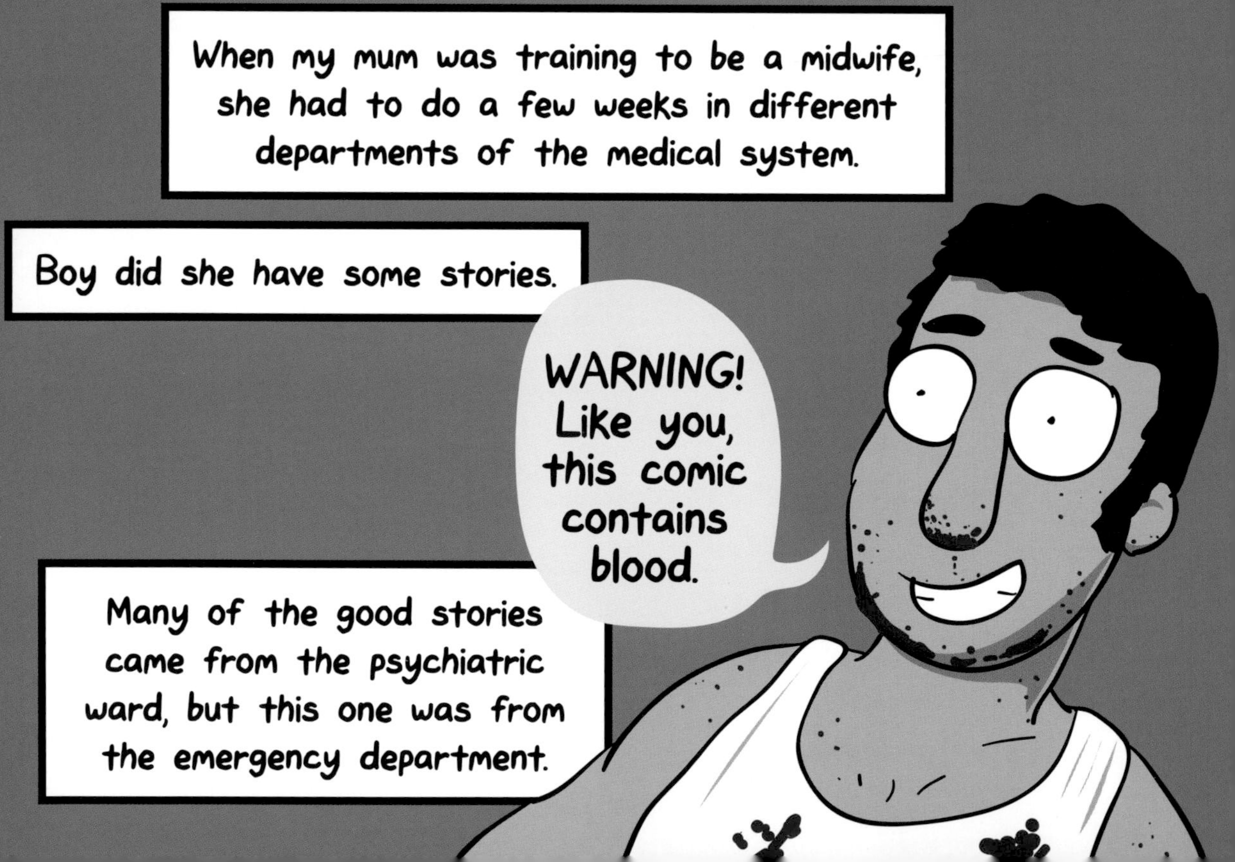

When my mum was training to be a midwife, she had to do a few weeks in different departments of the medical system.

Boy did she have some stories.

WARNING! Like you, this comic contains blood.

Many of the good stories came from the psychiatric ward, but this one was from the emergency department.

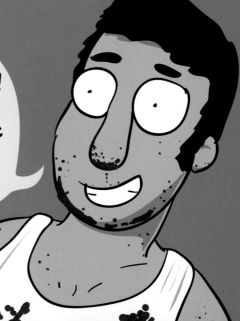

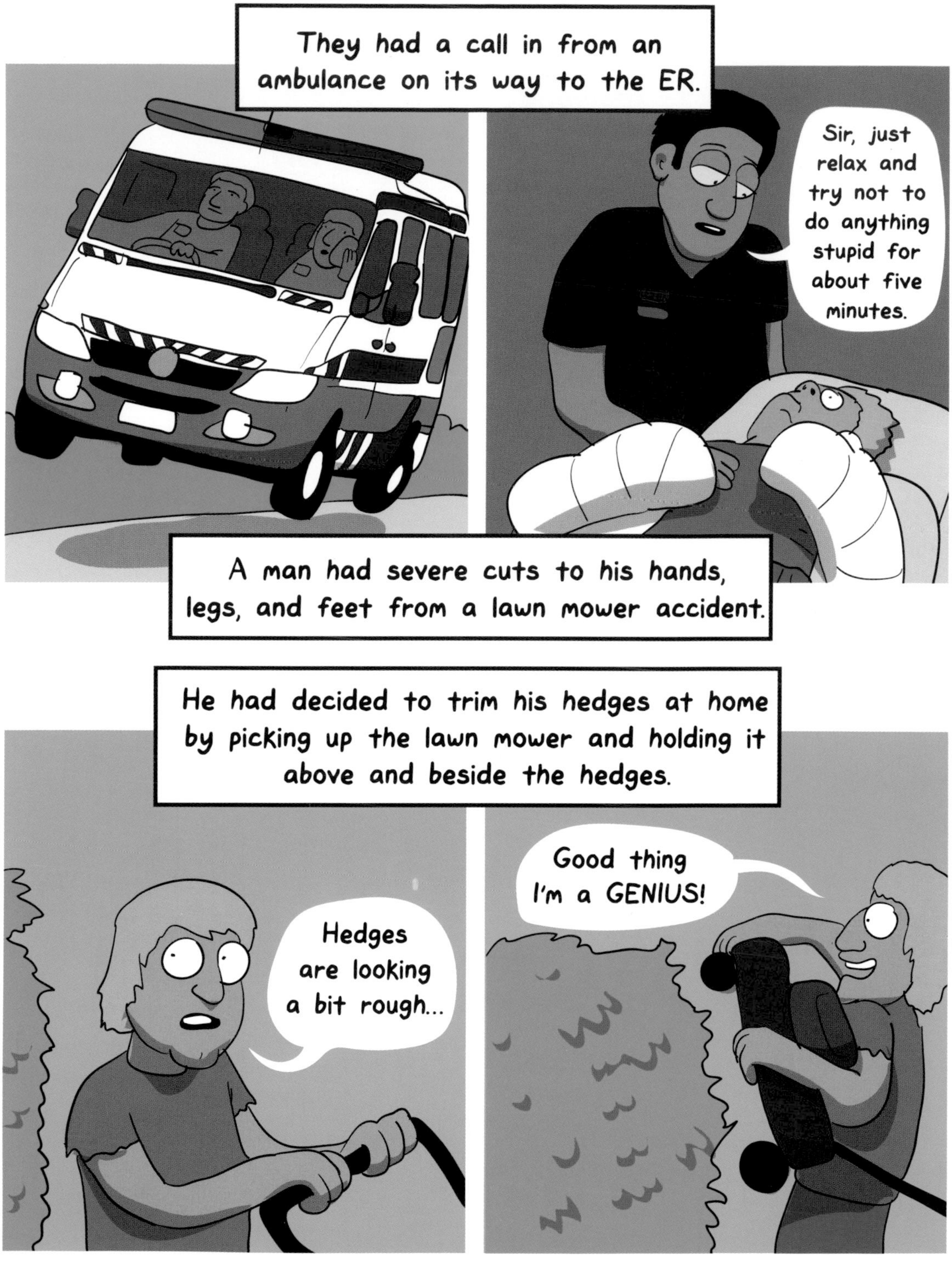
They had a call in from an ambulance on its way to the ER.
Sir, just relax and try not to do anything stupid for about five minutes.
A man had severe cuts to his hands, legs, and feet from a lawn mower accident.
He had decided to trim his hedges at home by picking up the lawn mower and holding it above and beside the hedges.
Hedges are looking a bit rough...
Good thing I'm a GENIUS!

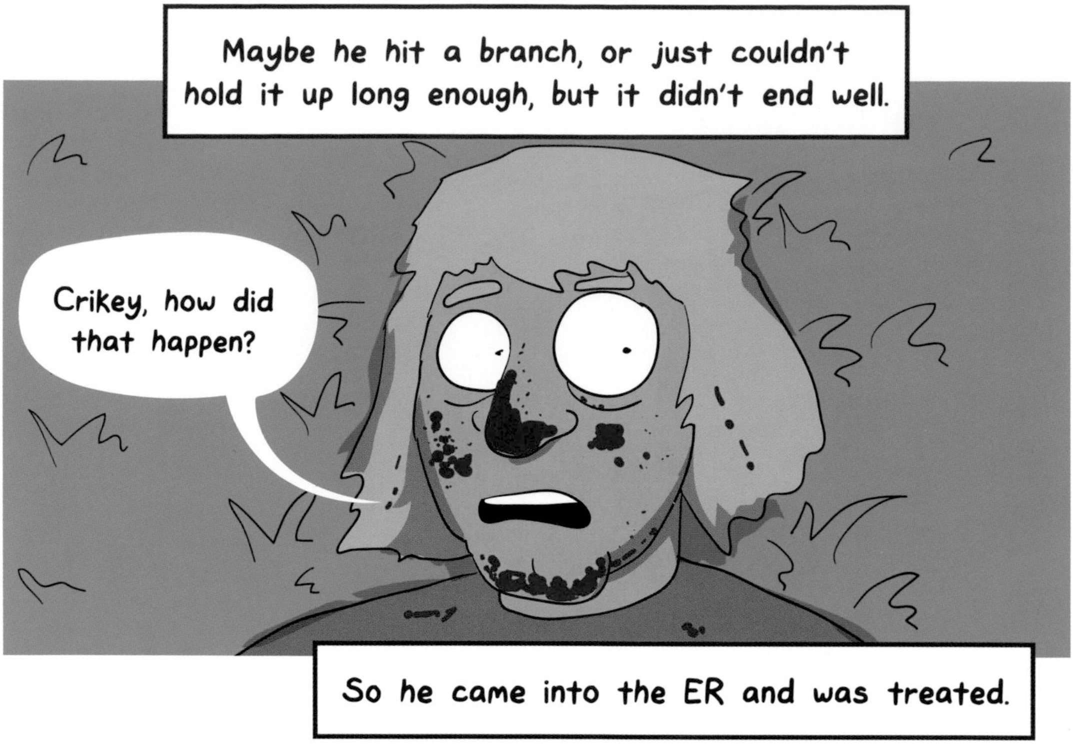
Maybe he hit a branch, or just couldn't hold it up long enough, but it didn't end well.
Crikey, how did that happen?
So he came into the ER and was treated.

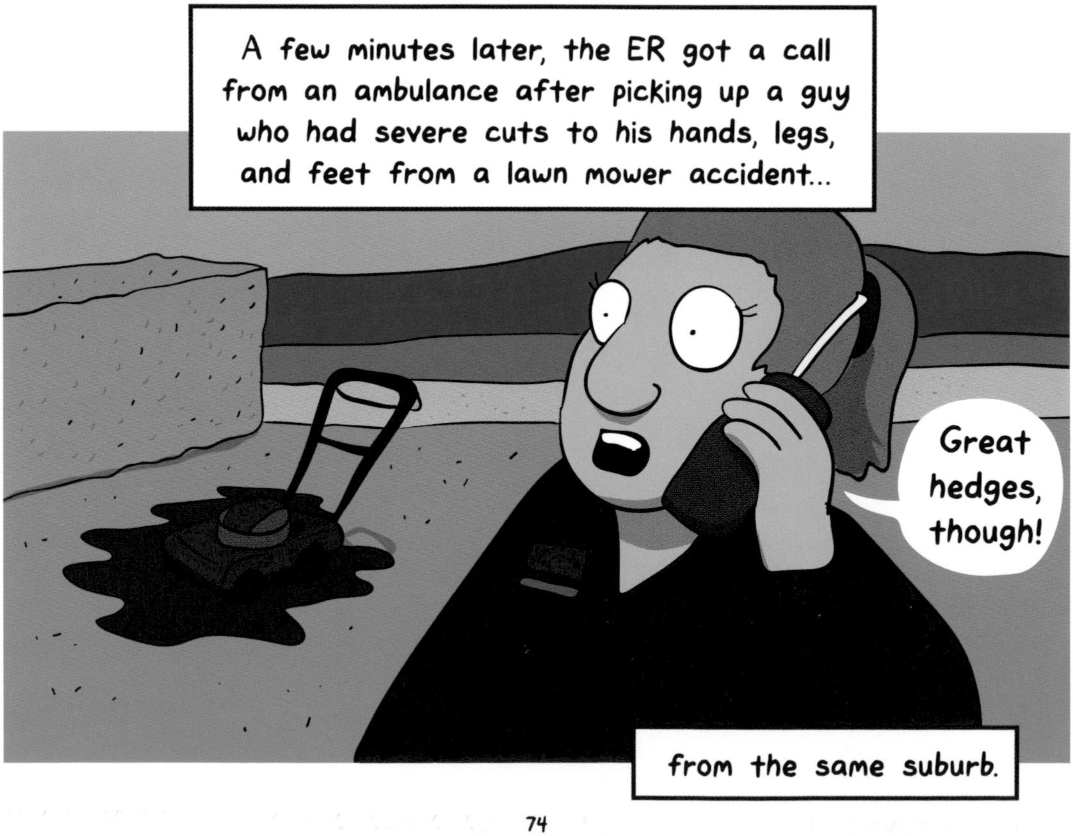
A few minutes later, the ER got a call from an ambulance after picking up a guy who had severe cuts to his hands, legs, and feet from a lawn mower accident...
Great hedges, though!
from the same suburb.

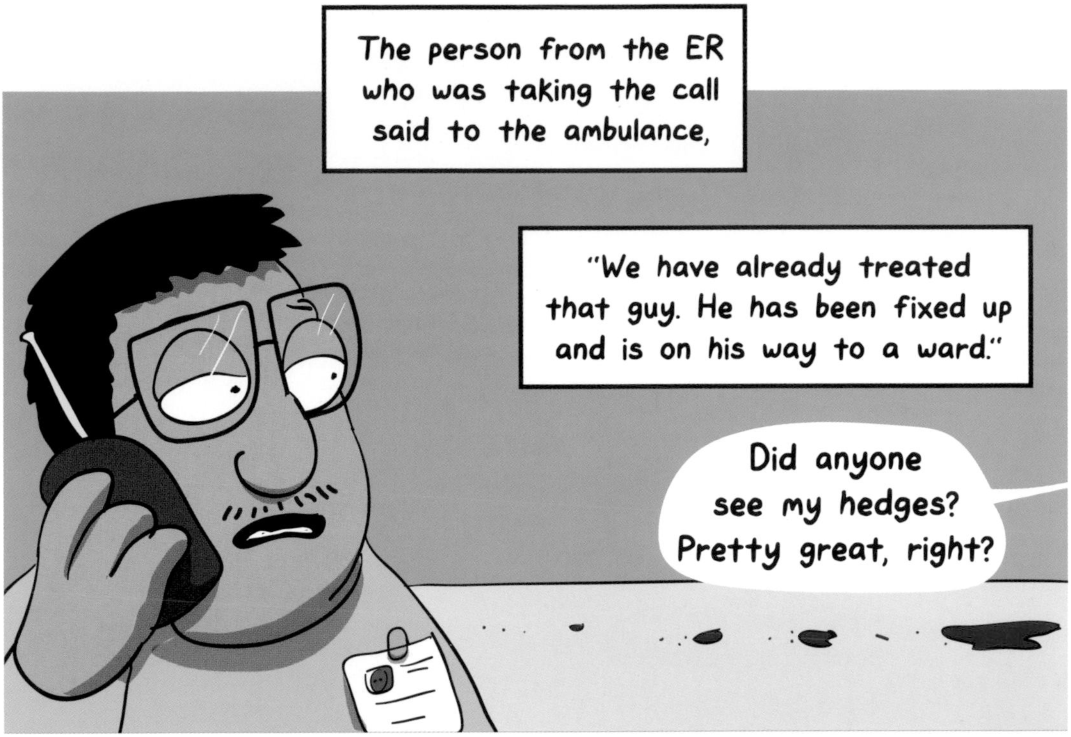
The person from the ER who was taking the call said to the ambulance,
"We have already treated that guy. He has been fixed up and is on his way to a ward."
Did anyone see my hedges? Pretty great, right?

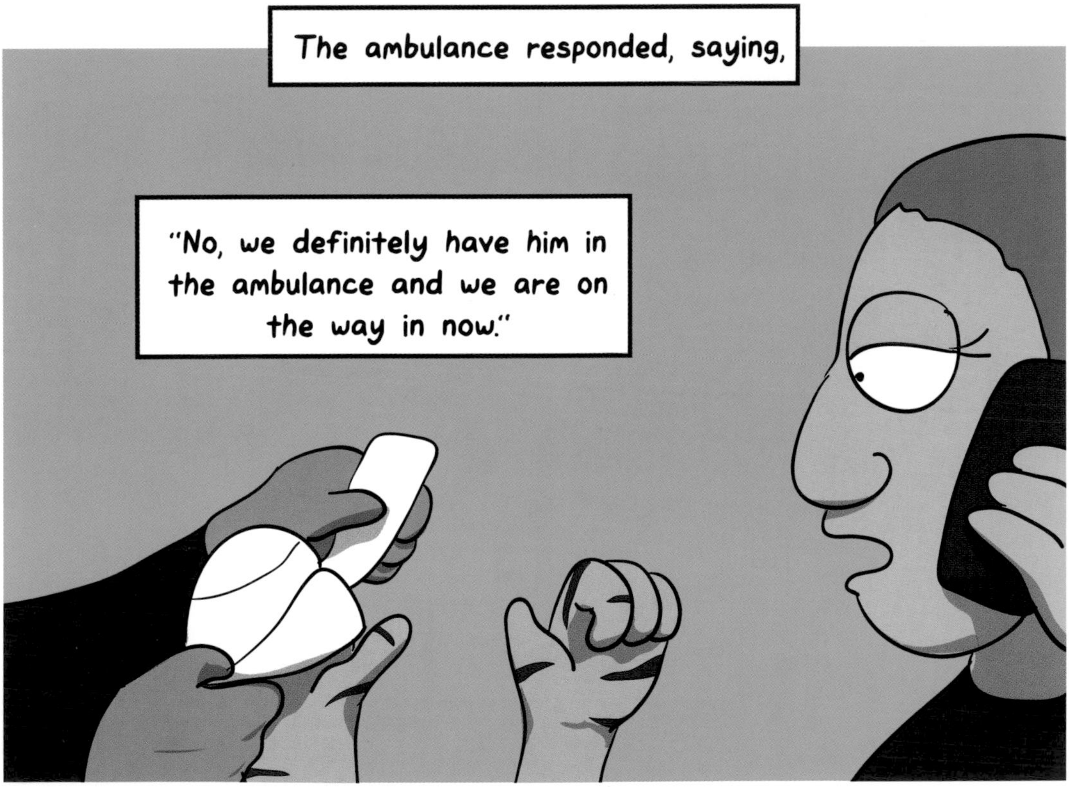
The ambulance responded, saying,
"No, we definitely have him in the ambulance and we are on the way in now."

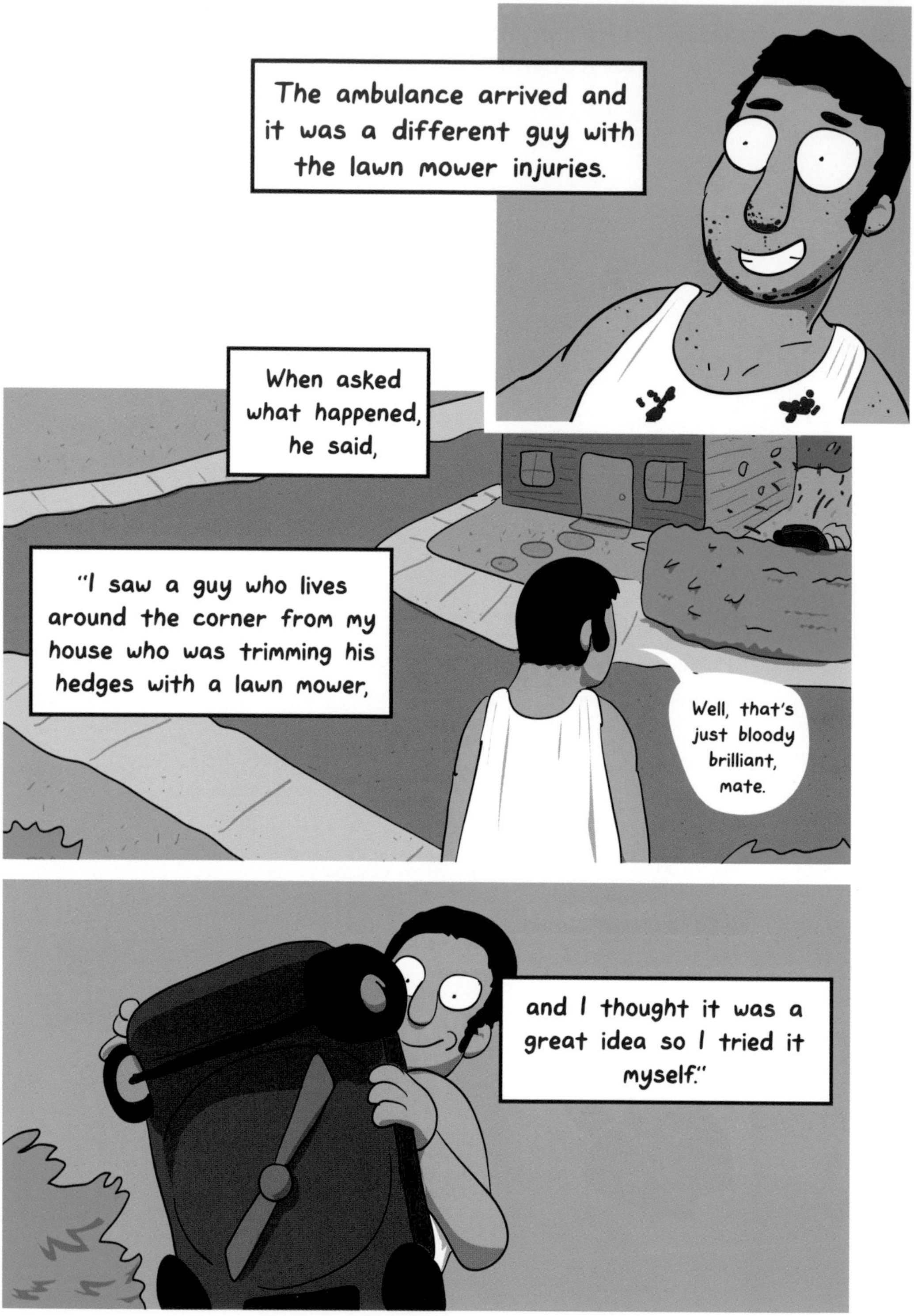
The ambulance arrived and it was a different guy with the lawn mower injuries.
When asked what happened, he said,
"I saw a guy who lives around the corner from my house who was trimming his hedges with a lawn mower,
Well, that's just bloody brilliant, mate.
and I thought it was a great idea so I tried it myself."

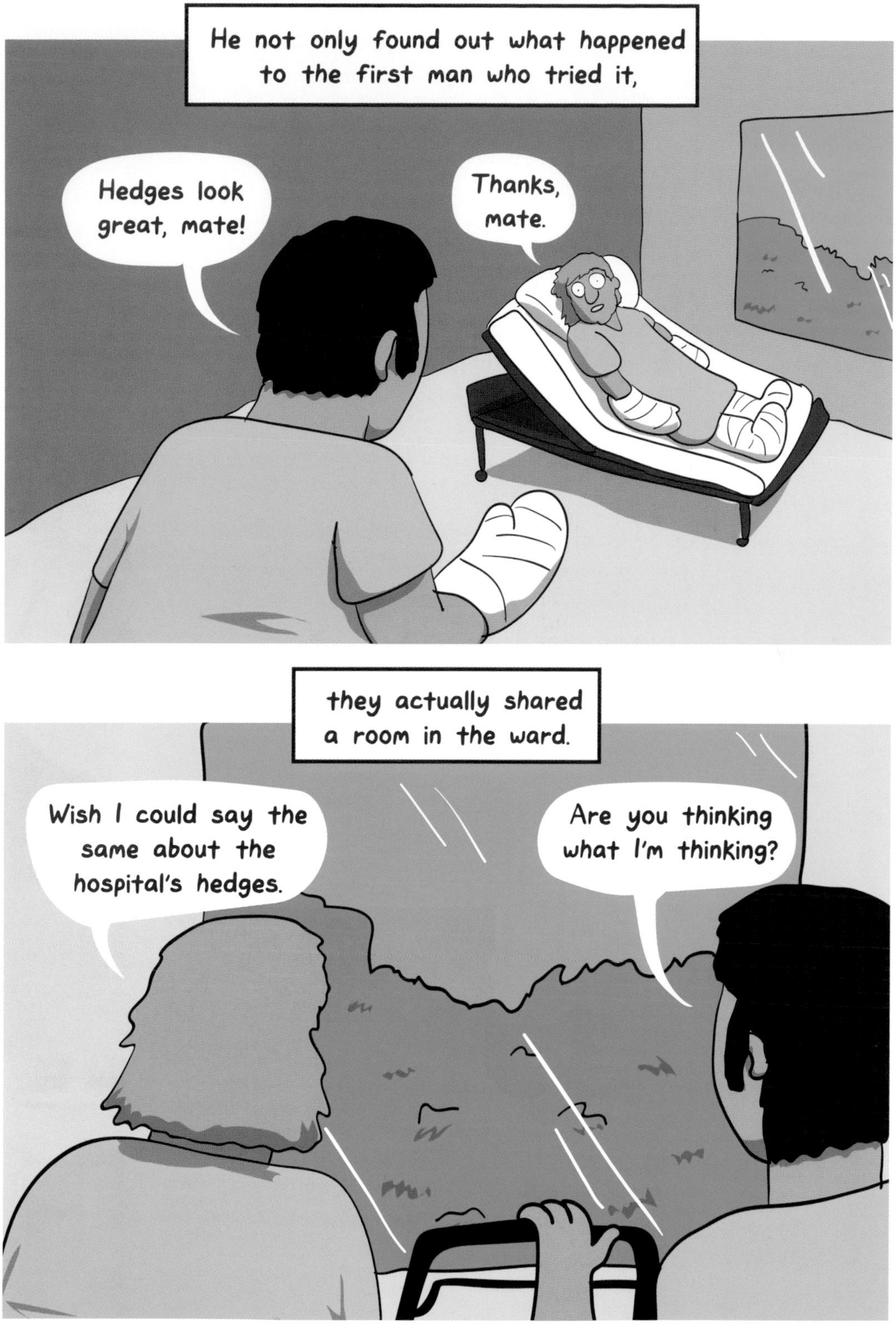
He not only found out what happened to the first man who tried it,
Hedges look great, mate!
Thanks, mate.
they actually shared a room in the ward.
Wish I could say the same about the hospital's hedges.
Are you thinking what I'm thinking?

# CHAPTER 12

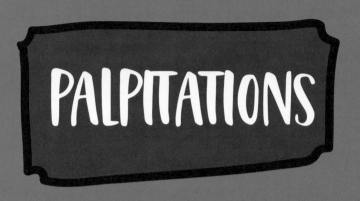

## PALPITATIONS

told by Kat R

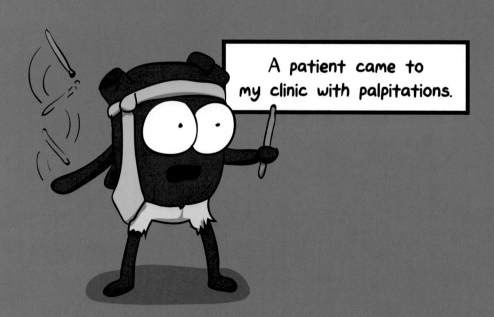

A patient came to my clinic with palpitations.

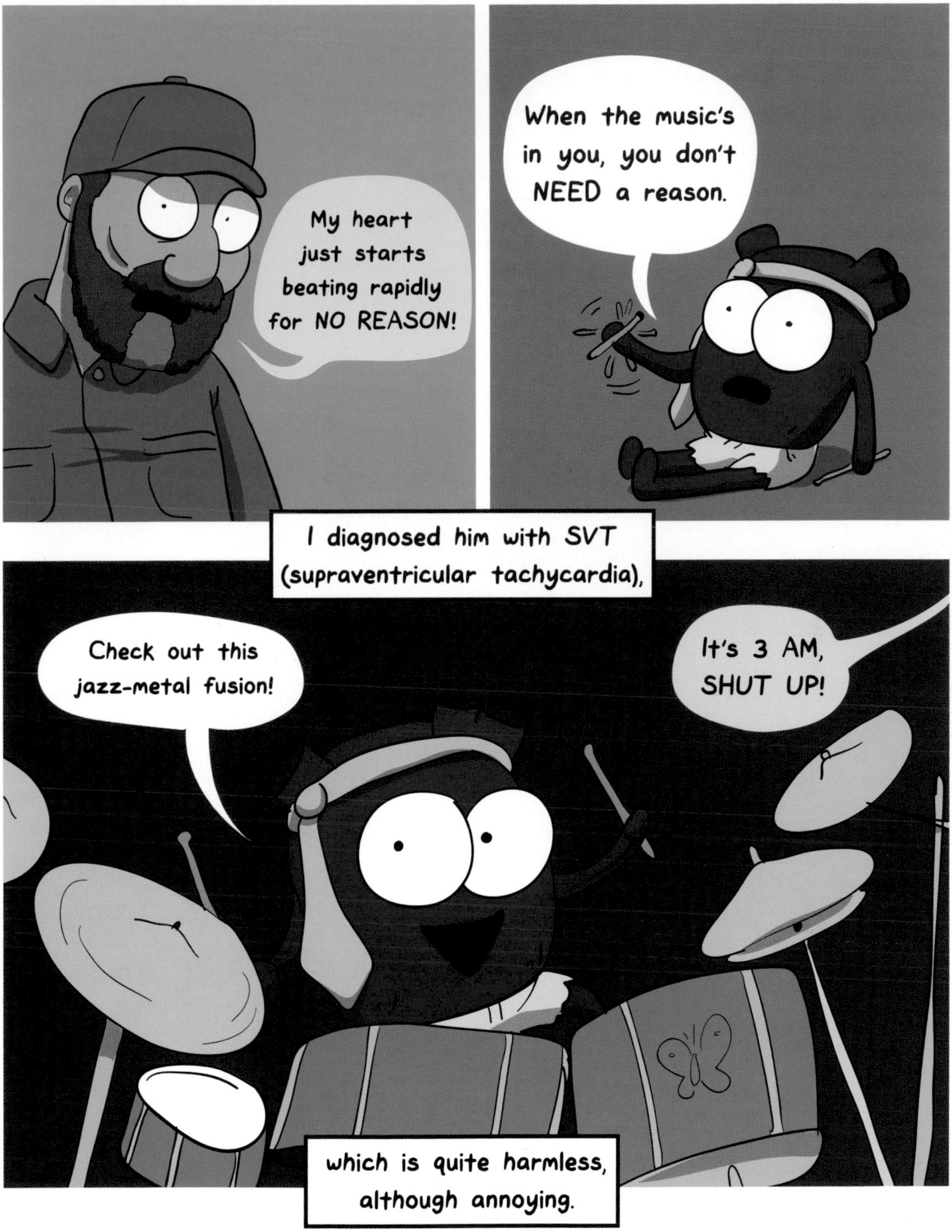
My heart just starts beating rapidly for NO REASON!
When the music's in you, you don't NEED a reason.
I diagnosed him with SVT (supraventricular tachycardia),
Check out this jazz-metal fusion!
It's 3 AM, SHUT UP!
which is quite harmless, although annoying.

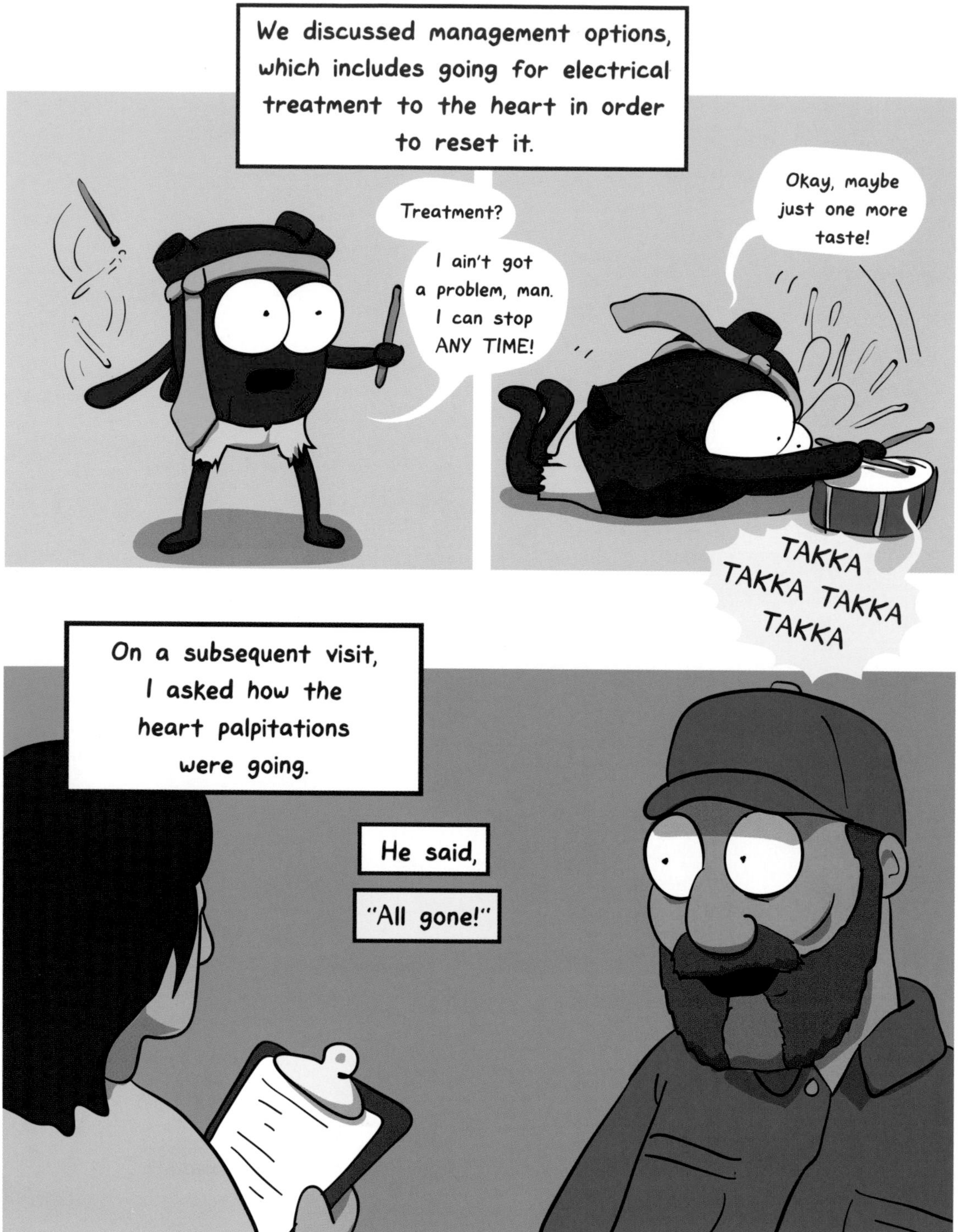
We discussed management options, which includes going for electrical treatment to the heart in order to reset it.
Treatment?
I ain't got a problem, man. I can stop ANY TIME!
Okay, maybe just one more taste!
TAKKA TAKKA TAKKA TAKKA
On a subsequent visit, I asked how the heart palpitations were going.
He said,
"All gone!"

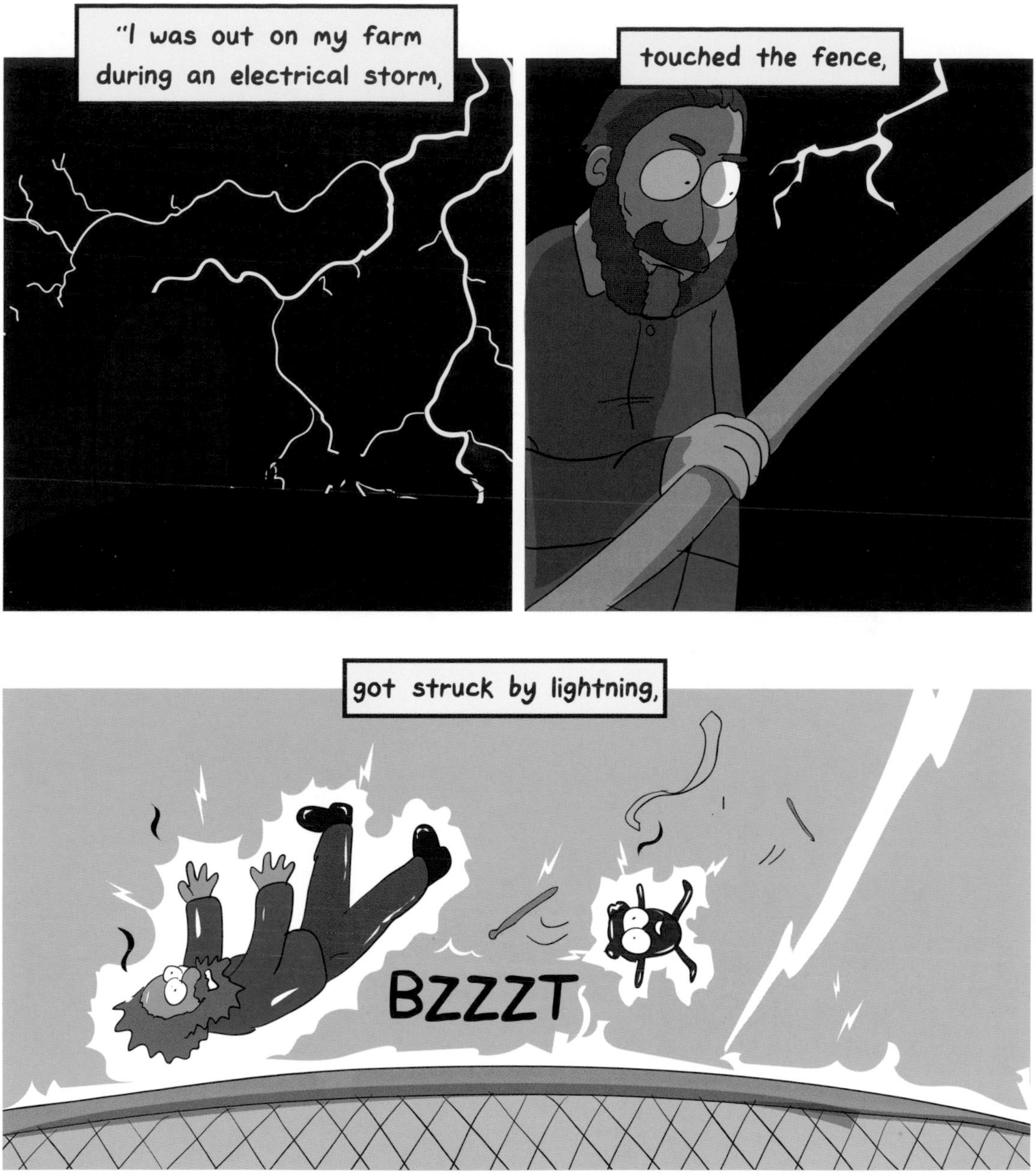
"I was out on my farm during an electrical storm,
touched the fence,
got struck by lightning,
BZZZT

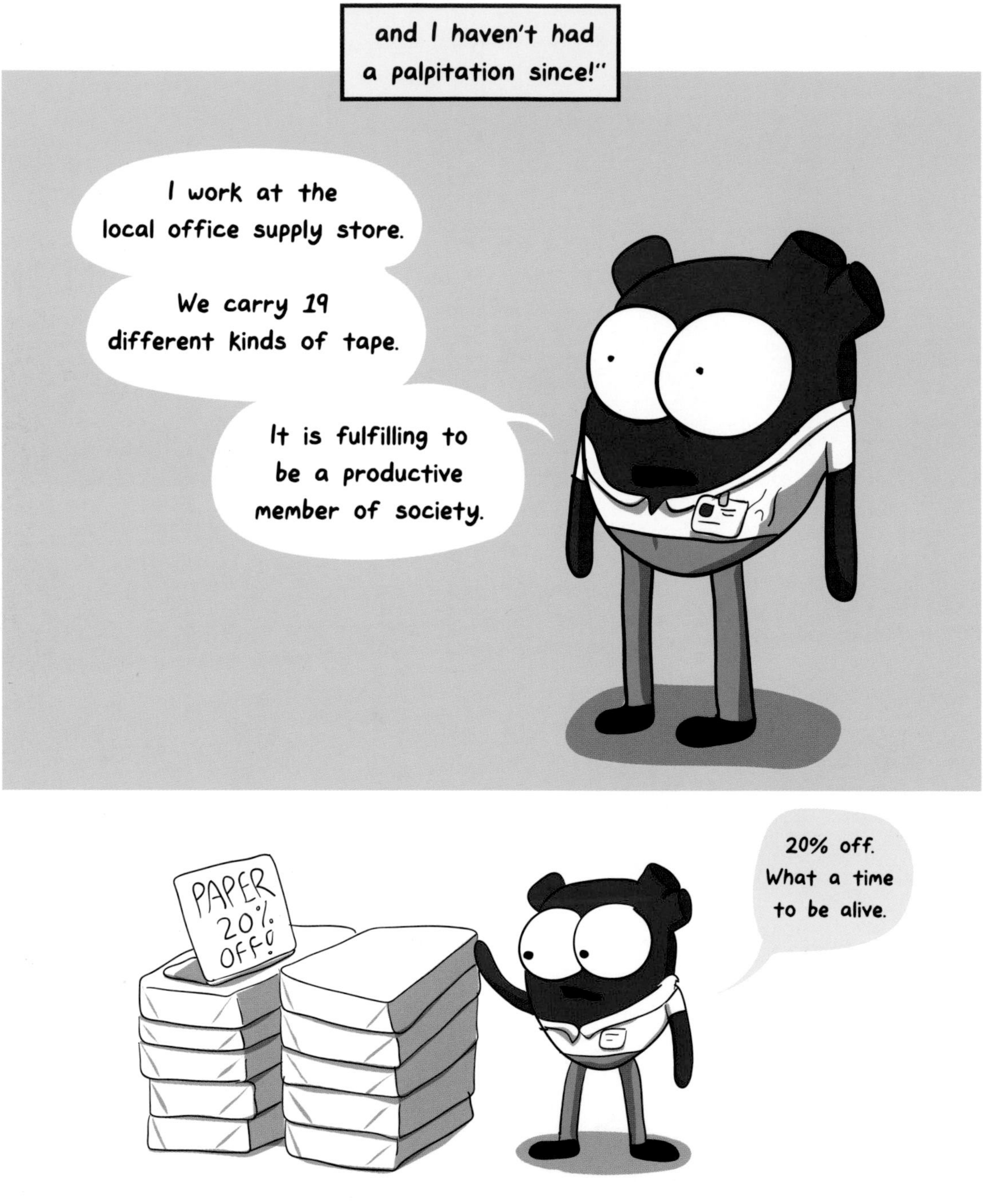
and I haven't had a palpitation since!"
I work at the local office supply store.
We carry 19 different kinds of tape.
It is fulfilling to be a productive member of society.
PAPER 20% OFF!
20% off. What a time to be alive.

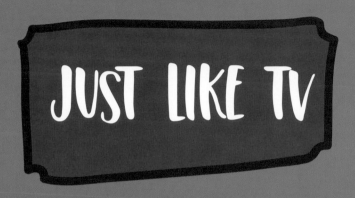

# CHAPTER 13

# JUST LIKE TV

## told by Dee

As a medical student, a question that people ask me all the time is whether working in a hospital is "just like on TV."

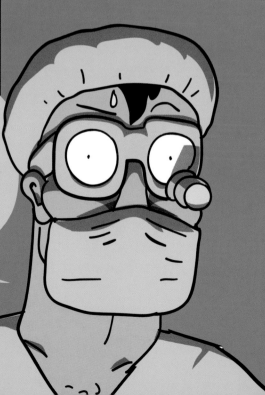

Twenty CCs of DRAMA, STAT!

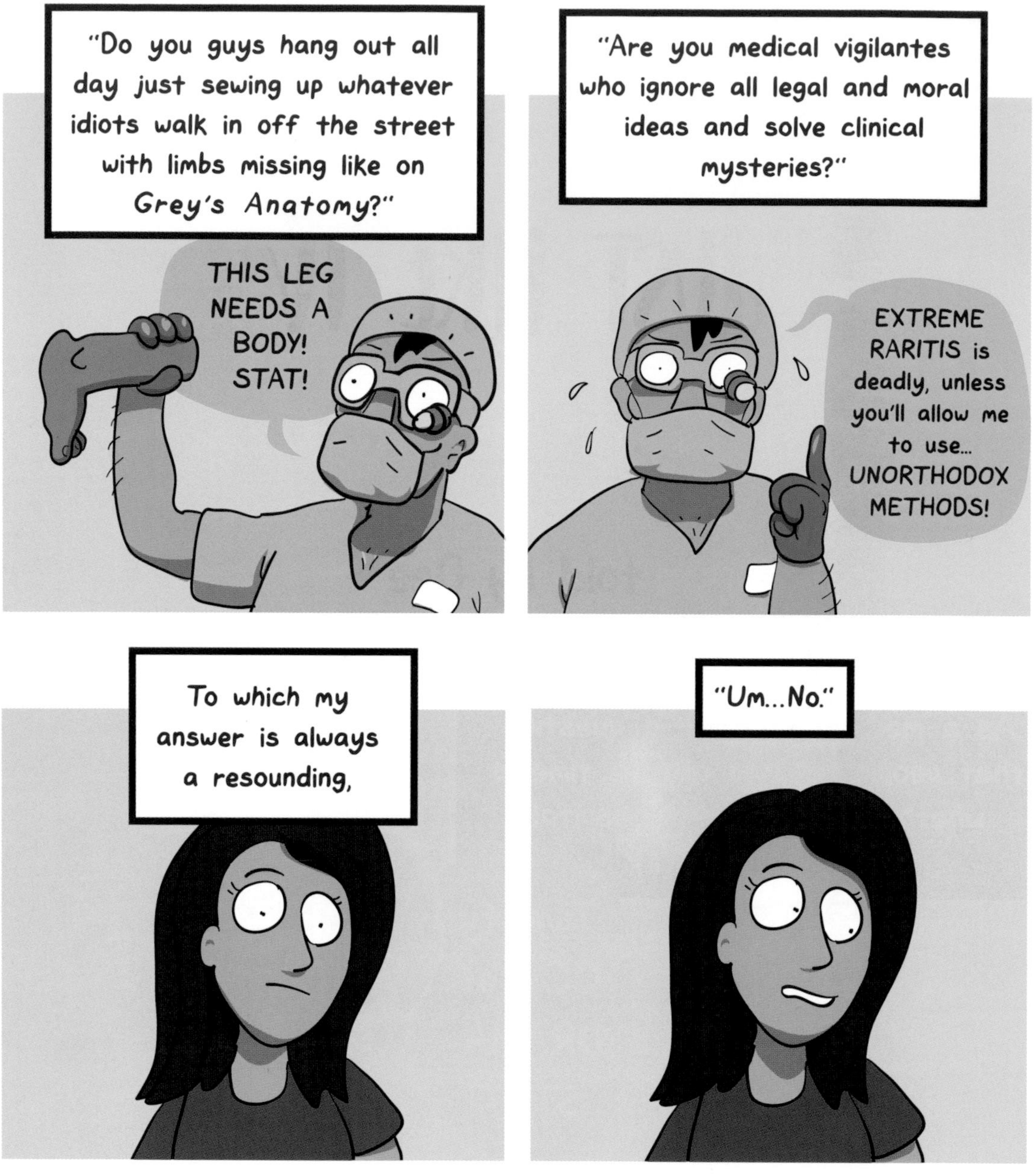
"Do you guys hang out all day just sewing up whatever idiots walk in off the street with limbs missing like on Grey's Anatomy?"
THIS LEG NEEDS A BODY! STAT!
"Are you medical vigilantes who ignore all legal and moral ideas and solve clinical mysteries?"
EXTREME RARITIS is deadly, unless you'll allow me to use... UNORTHODOX METHODS!
To which my answer is always a resounding,
"Um...No."

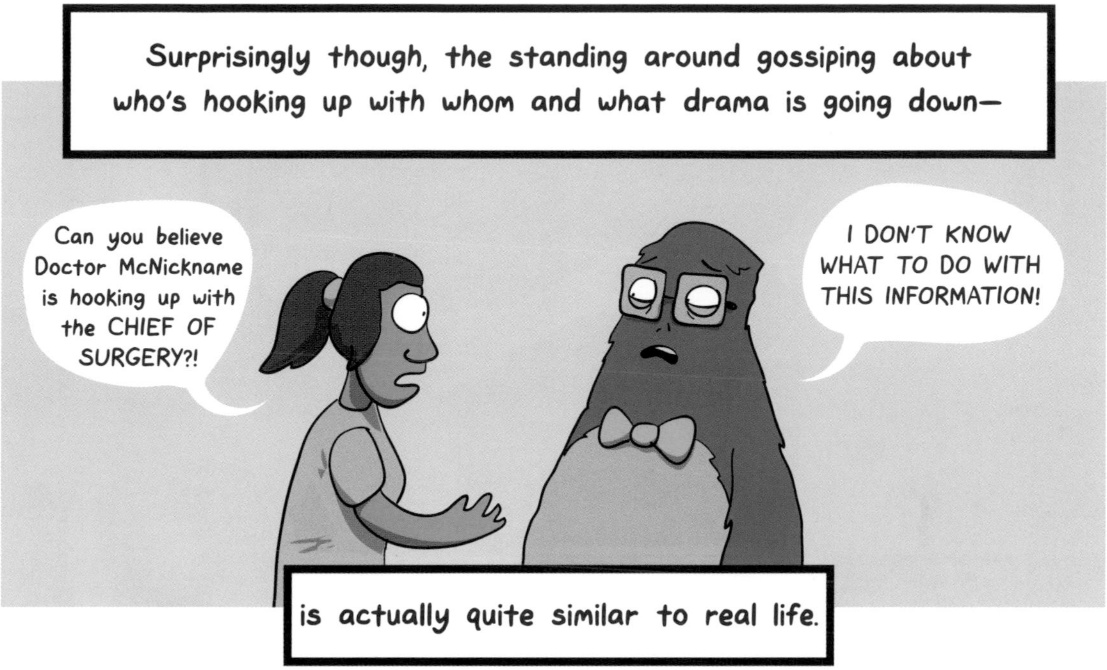

Surprisingly though, the standing around gossiping about who's hooking up with whom and what drama is going down—

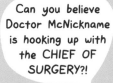

Can you believe Doctor McNickname is hooking up with the CHIEF OF SURGERY?!

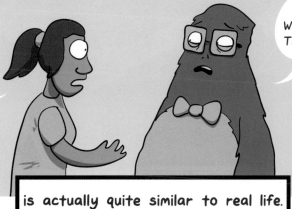

I DON'T KNOW WHAT TO DO WITH THIS INFORMATION!

is actually quite similar to real life.

I was on my Obstetrics and Gynecology rotation as a third-year medical student overnight in the Labor and Delivery floor. That's where all the babies are born.

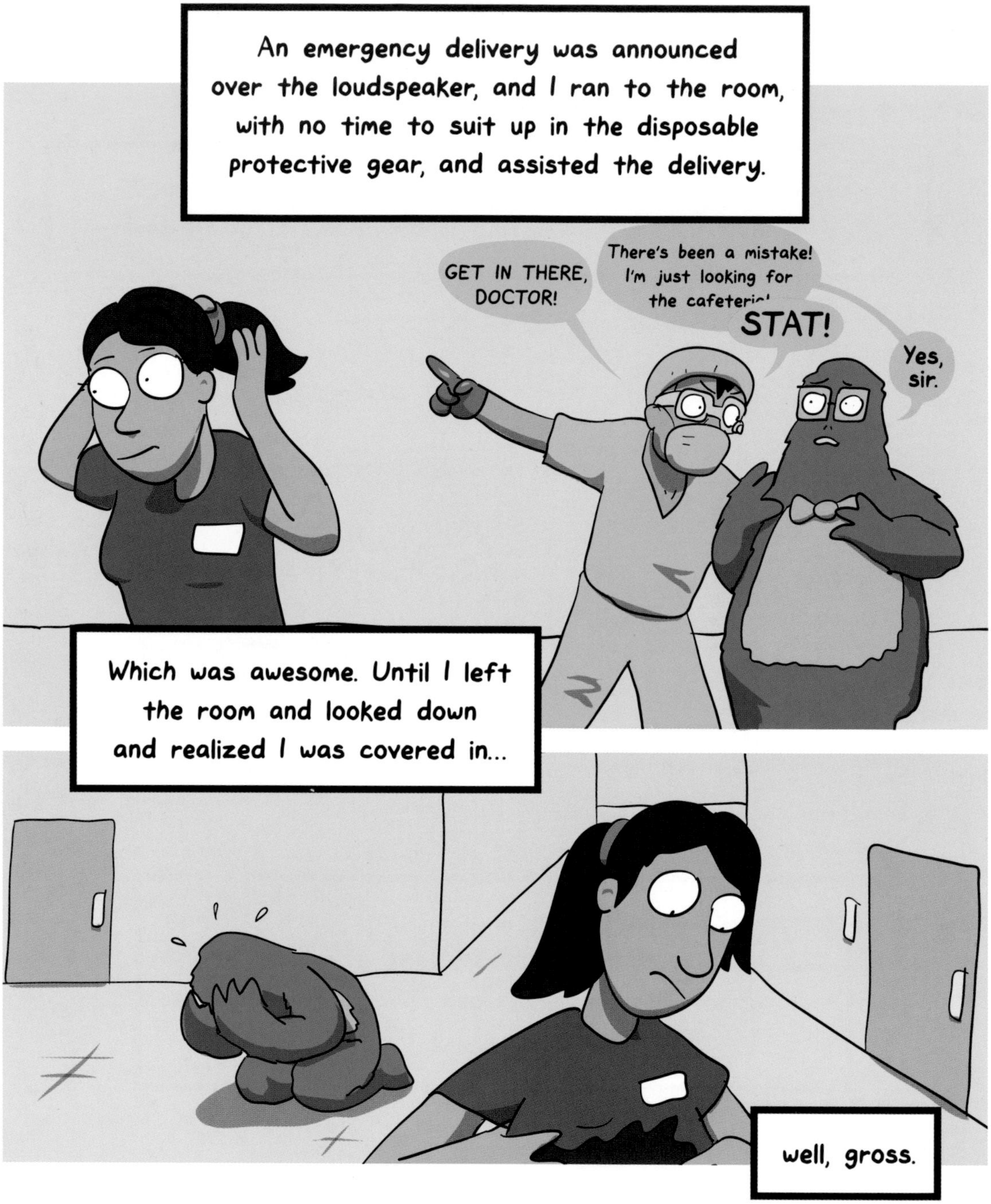
An emergency delivery was announced over the loudspeaker, and I ran to the room, with no time to suit up in the disposable protective gear, and assisted the delivery.
GET IN THERE, DOCTOR!
There's been a mistake! I'm just looking for the cafeteri-
STAT!
Yes, sir.
Which was awesome. Until I left the room and looked down and realized I was covered in...
well, gross.

We get our scrubs from a vending machine in the hospital.

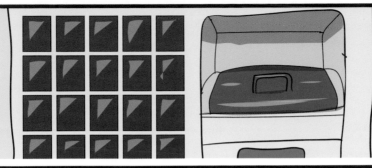

You only have a certain amount of credits,
and you have to return a set before you get it back.

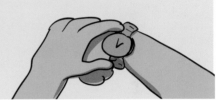

I had zero credits left on my card,

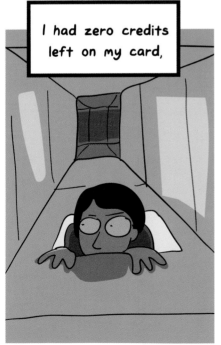

which meant if I wanted a clean set, I needed to put the pair I was wearing into the machine.

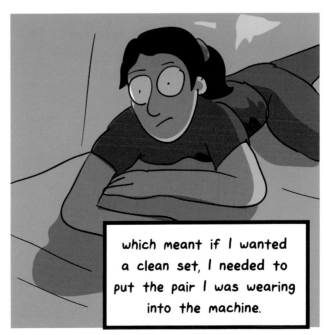

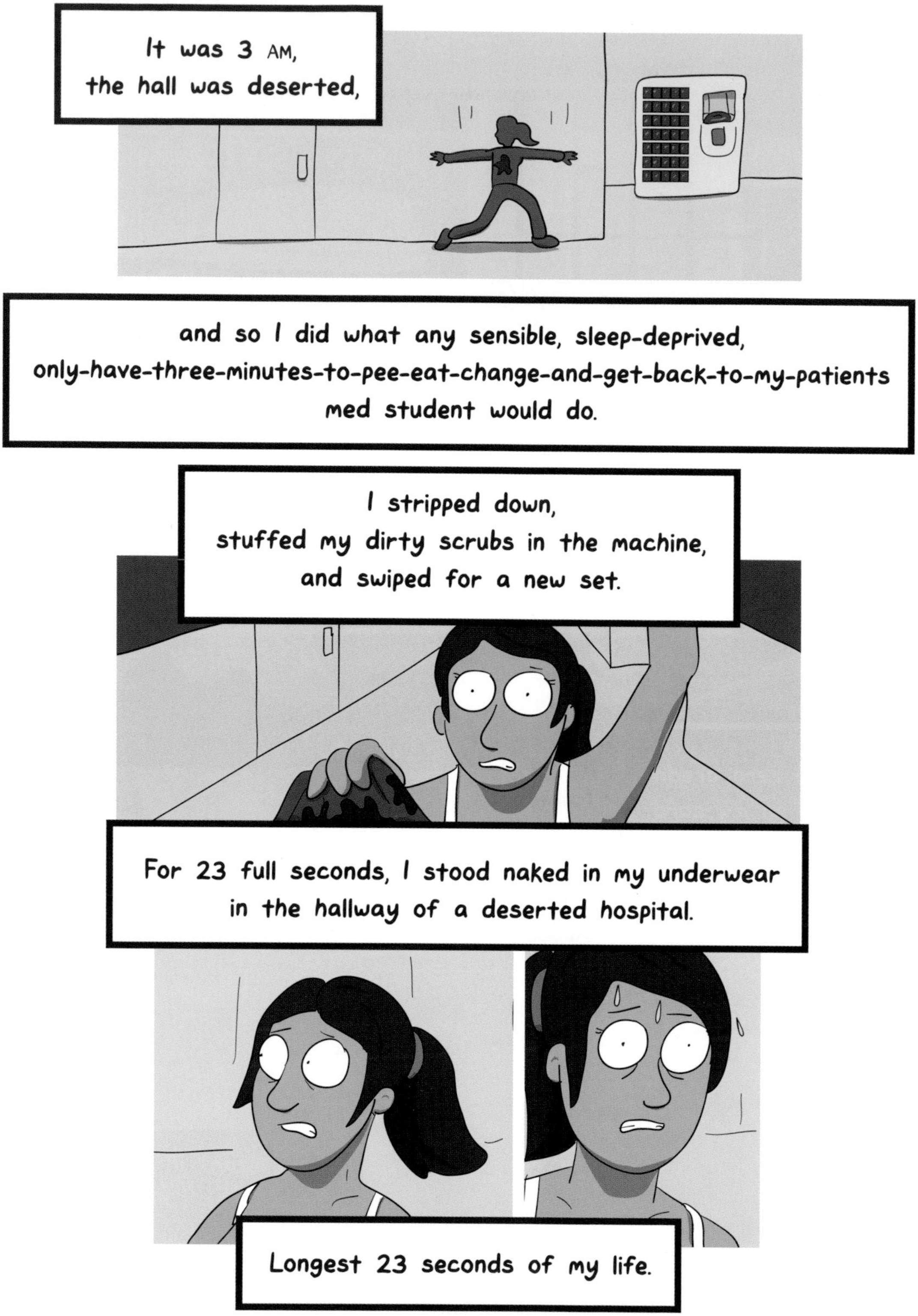
It was 3 AM,
the hall was deserted,
and so I did what any sensible, sleep-deprived, only-have-three-minutes-to-pee-eat-change-and-get-back-to-my-patients med student would do.
I stripped down, stuffed my dirty scrubs in the machine, and swiped for a new set.
For 23 full seconds, I stood naked in my underwear in the hallway of a deserted hospital.
Longest 23 seconds of my life.

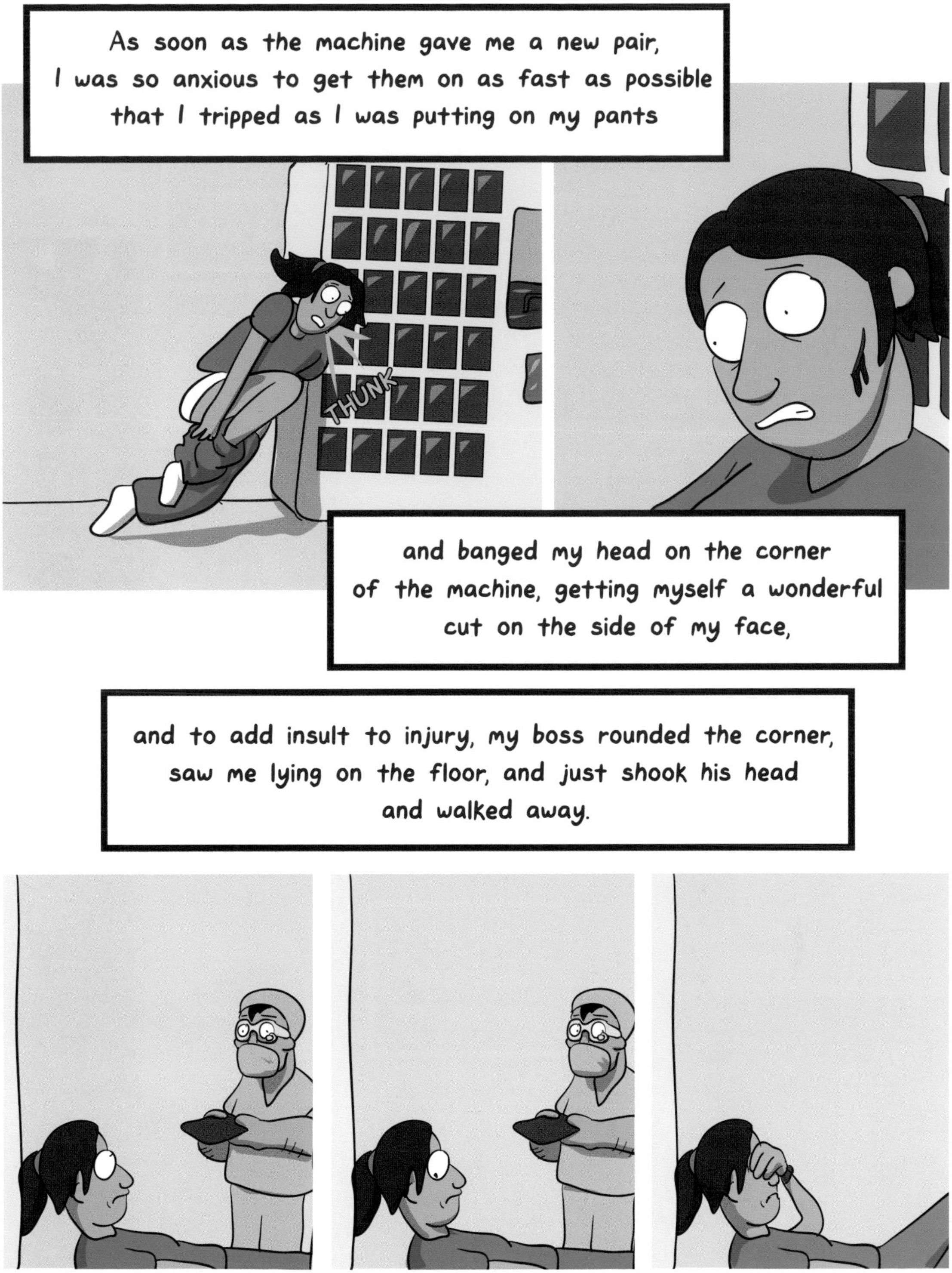
As soon as the machine gave me a new pair, I was so anxious to get them on as fast as possible that I tripped as I was putting on my pants
THUNK
and banged my head on the corner of the machine, getting myself a wonderful cut on the side of my face,
and to add insult to injury, my boss rounded the corner, saw me lying on the floor, and just shook his head and walked away.

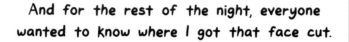

And for the rest of the night, everyone wanted to know where I got that face cut.

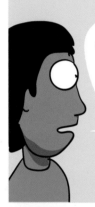

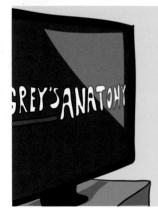

Wow, since you're a doctor, like on TV, I bet you got that from restraining a belligerent patient!

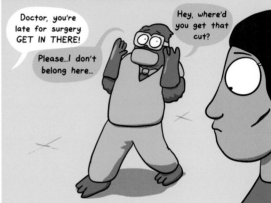

Doctor, you're late for surgery GET IN THERE!

Please...I don't belong here...

Hey, where'd you get that cut?

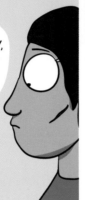

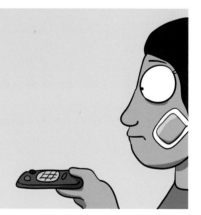

GREY'S ANATOMY

So yes, my life is just like TV.

CHAPTER 14

# POPCORN

told by Colin

I used to love popcorn.

WARNING: Contains popcorn.

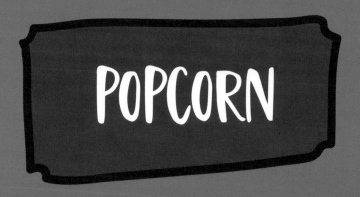

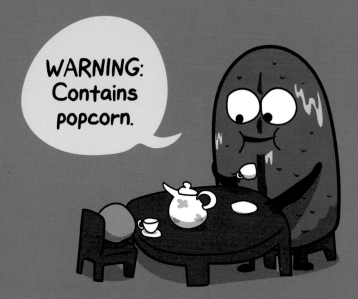

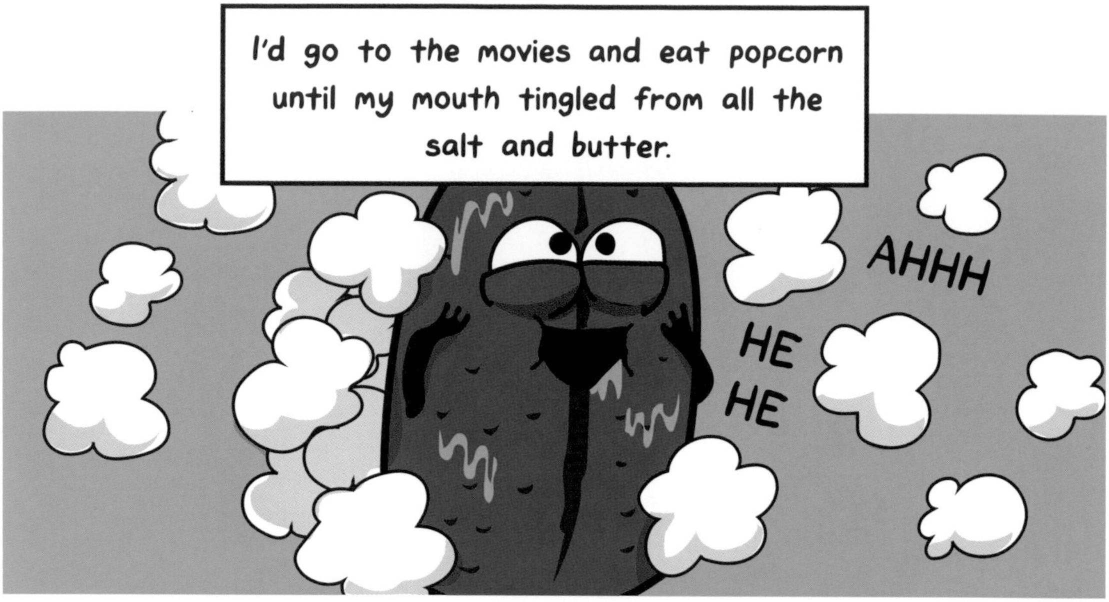
I'd go to the movies and eat popcorn until my mouth tingled from all the salt and butter.
AHHH
HE HE

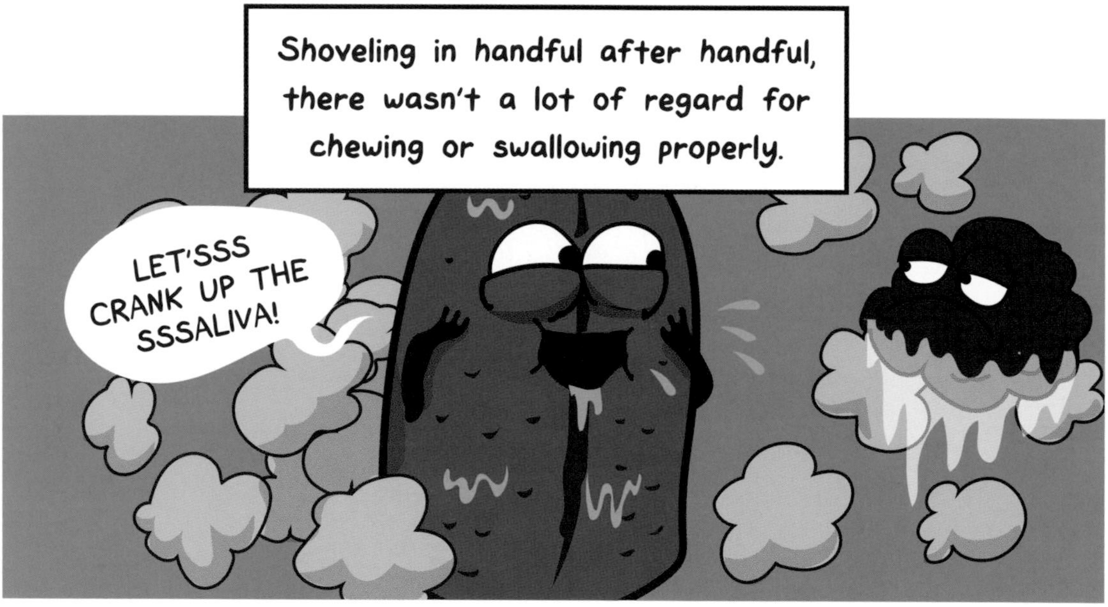
Shoveling in handful after handful, there wasn't a lot of regard for chewing or swallowing properly.
LET'SSS CRANK UP THE SSSALIVA!

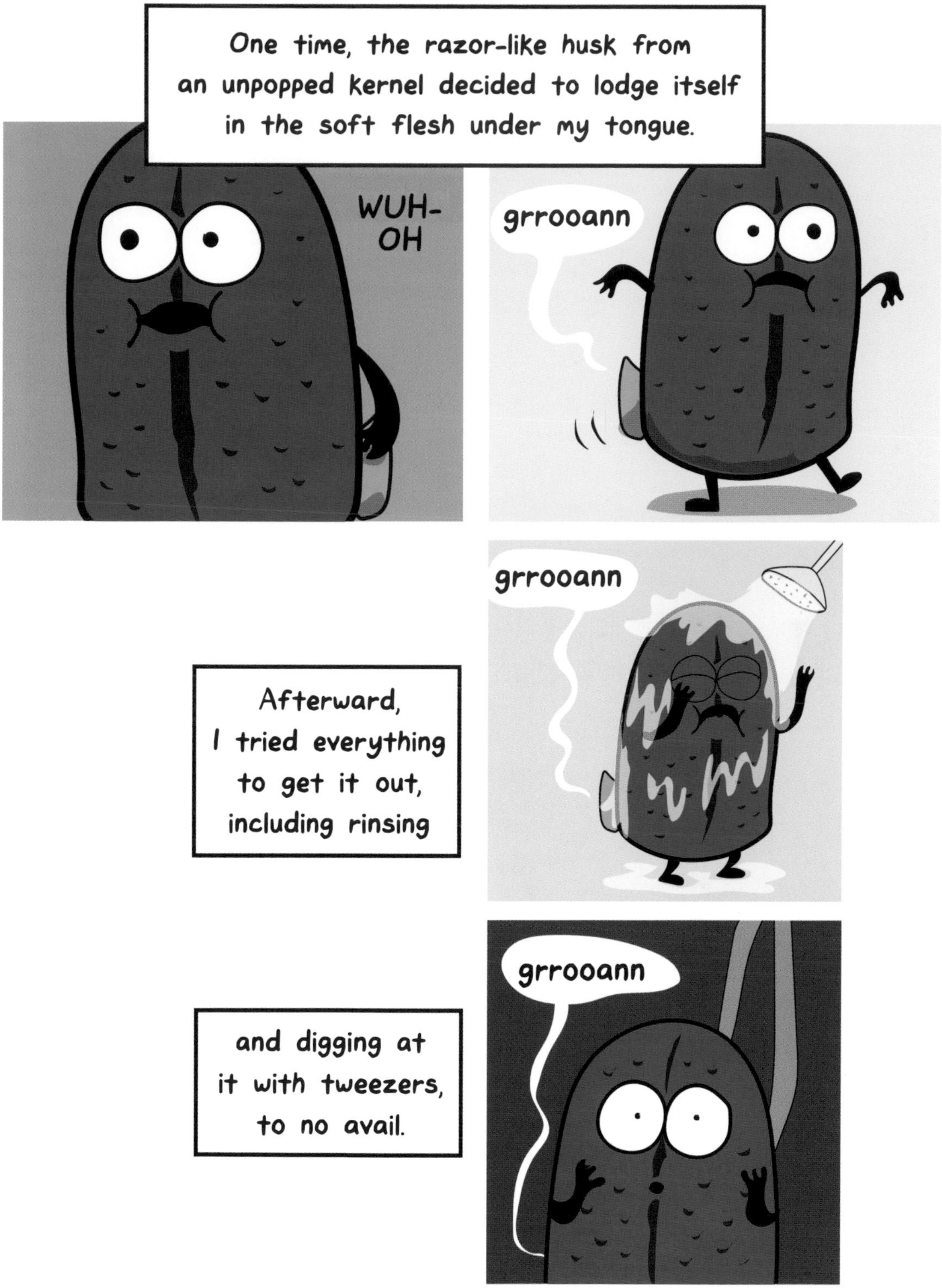
One time, the razor-like husk from an unpopped kernel decided to lodge itself in the soft flesh under my tongue.
WUH-OH
grrooann
grrooann
Afterward, I tried everything to get it out, including rinsing
grrooann
and digging at it with tweezers, to no avail.

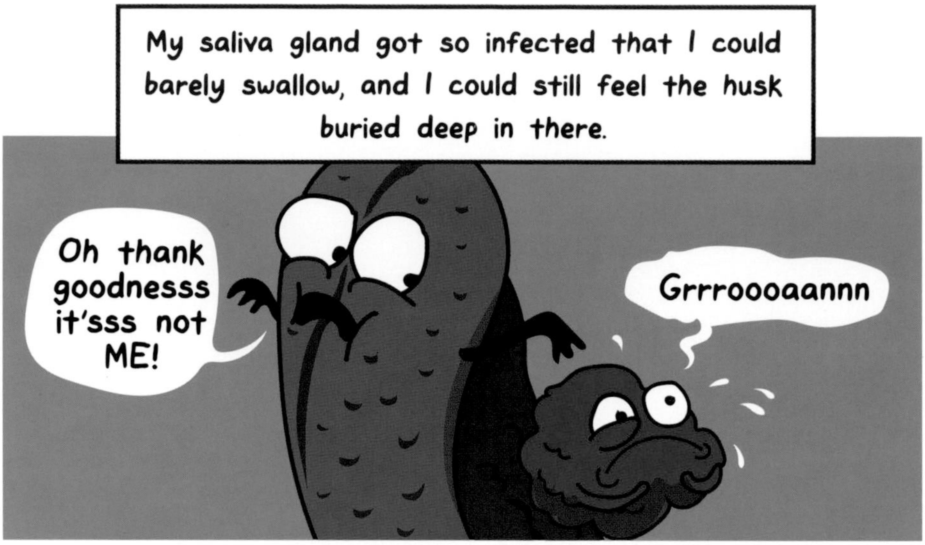
My saliva gland got so infected that I could barely swallow, and I could still feel the husk buried deep in there.
Oh thank goodnesss it'sss not ME!
Grrroooaannn

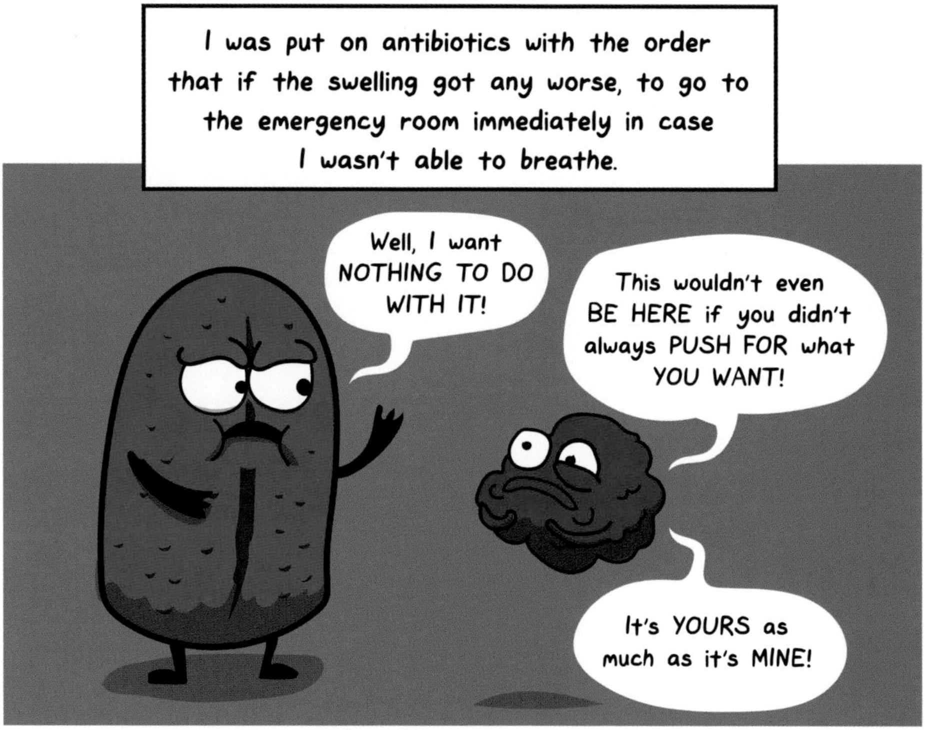
I was put on antibiotics with the order that if the swelling got any worse, to go to the emergency room immediately in case I wasn't able to breathe.
Well, I want NOTHING TO DO WITH IT!
This wouldn't even BE HERE if you didn't always PUSH FOR what YOU WANT!
It's YOURS as much as it's MINE!

You're inSATIABLE!
I admit it. I'm addicted to POPCORN!
GRROOOOAAAANN

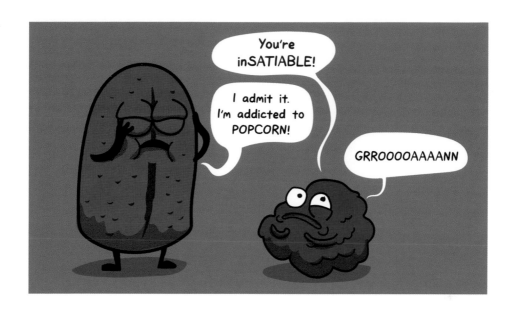

A day or two later, my saliva gland had become the size of a small football,

THAT'SS IT! WE'RE GETTING THISS THING OUT OF YOU!

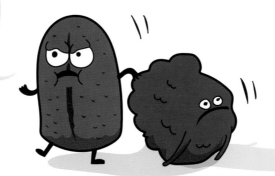

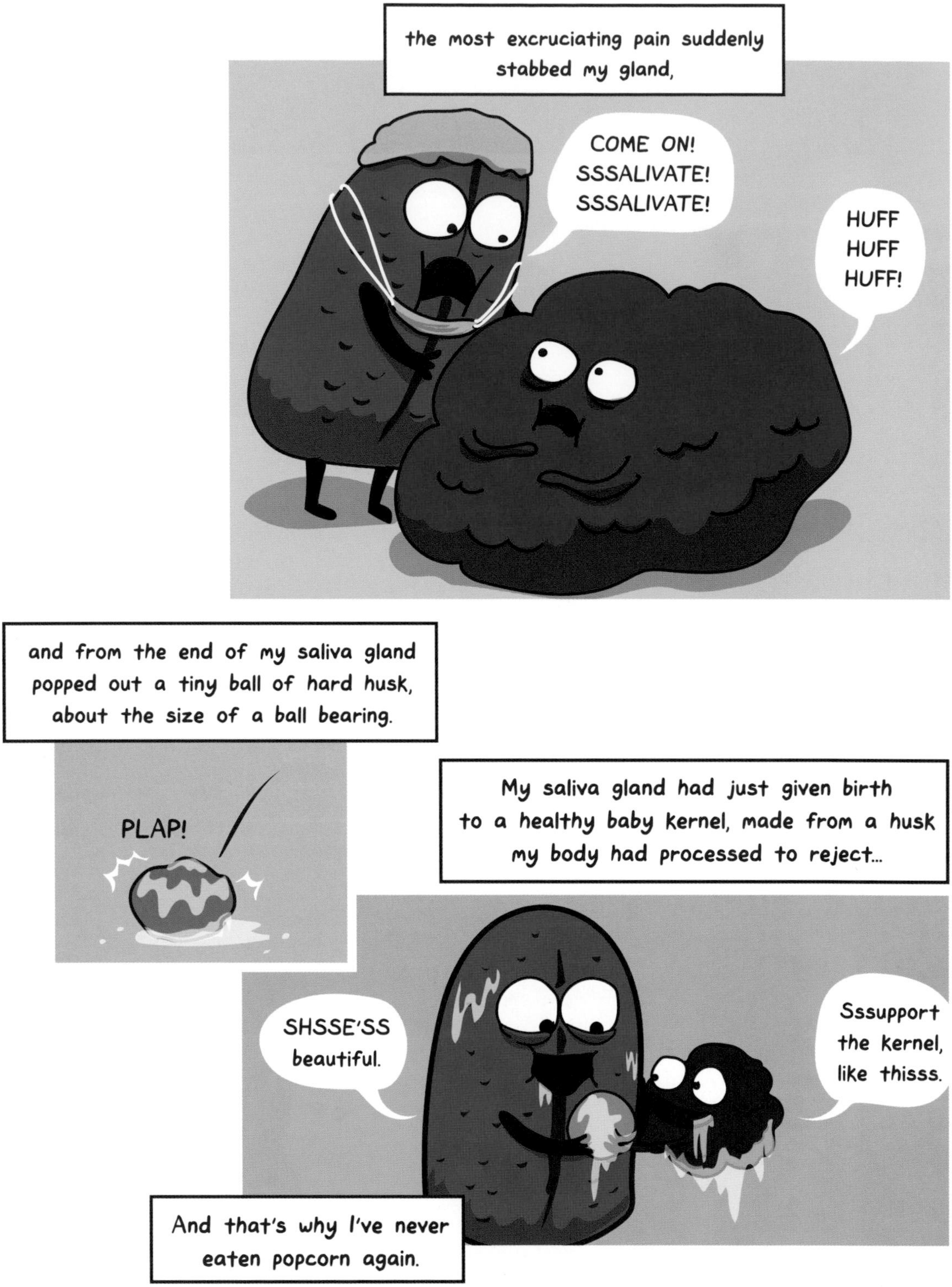
the most excruciating pain suddenly stabbed my gland,
COME ON! SSSALIVATE! SSSALIVATE!
HUFF HUFF HUFF!
and from the end of my saliva gland popped out a tiny ball of hard husk, about the size of a ball bearing.
PLAP!
My saliva gland had just given birth to a healthy baby kernel, made from a husk my body had processed to reject...
SHSSE'SS beautiful.
Sssupport the kernel, like thisss.
And that's why I've never eaten popcorn again.

CHAPTER 15

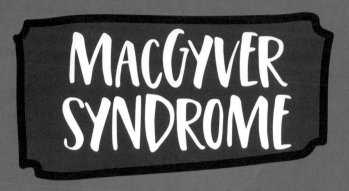

# MacGyver Syndrome

## told by MindfulAide

I have a friend who was a proctologist in California,
and we all know proctologists have the best medical stories...

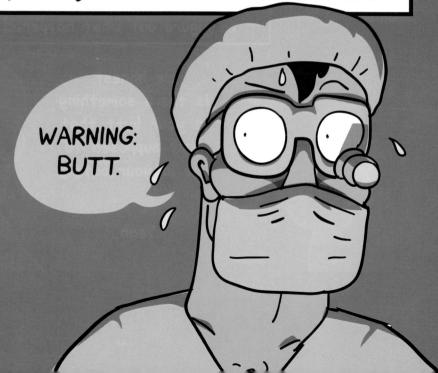

WARNING:
BUTT.

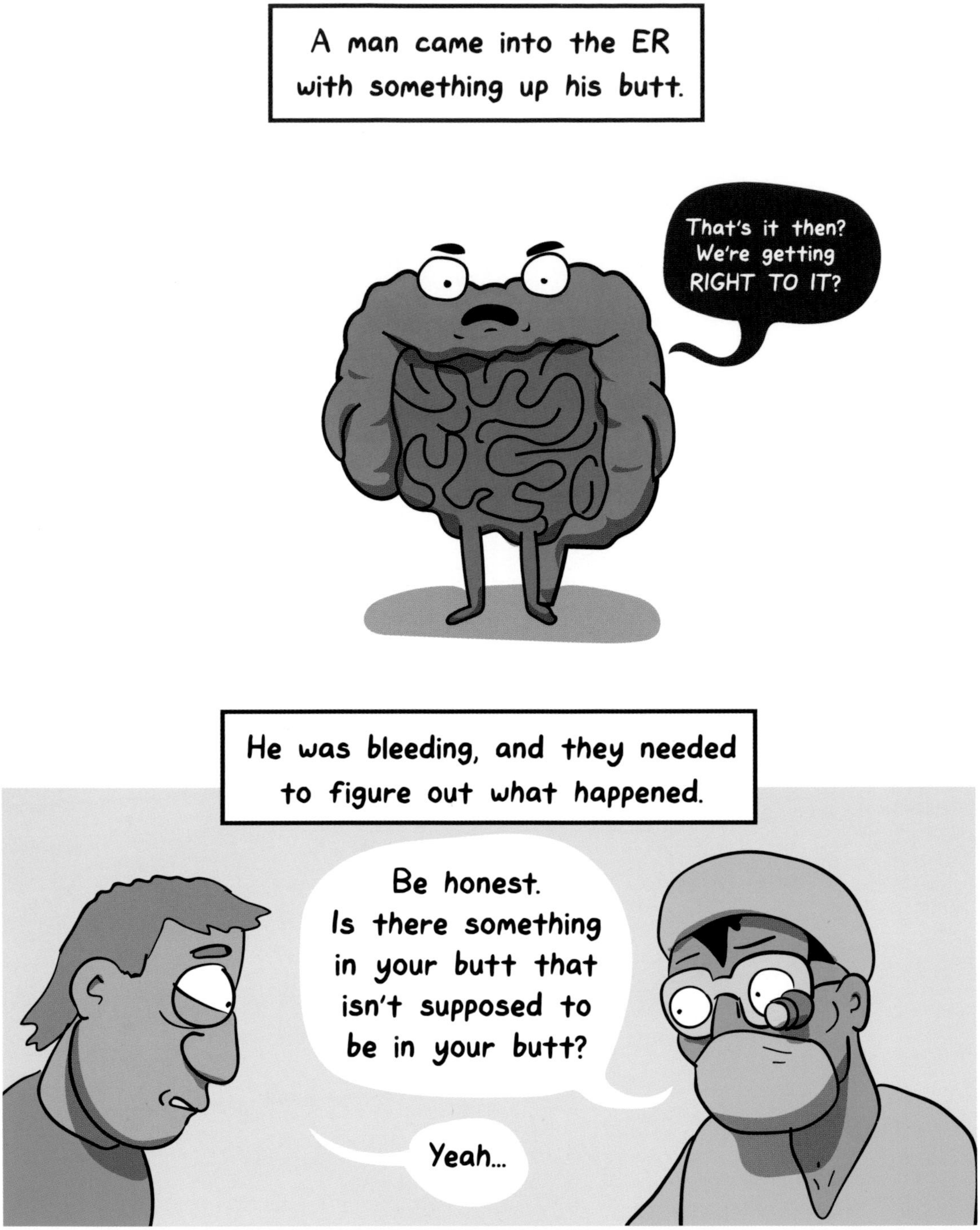
A man came into the ER with something up his butt.
That's it then? We're getting RIGHT TO IT?
He was bleeding, and they needed to figure out what happened.
Be honest. Is there something in your butt that isn't supposed to be in your butt?
Yeah...

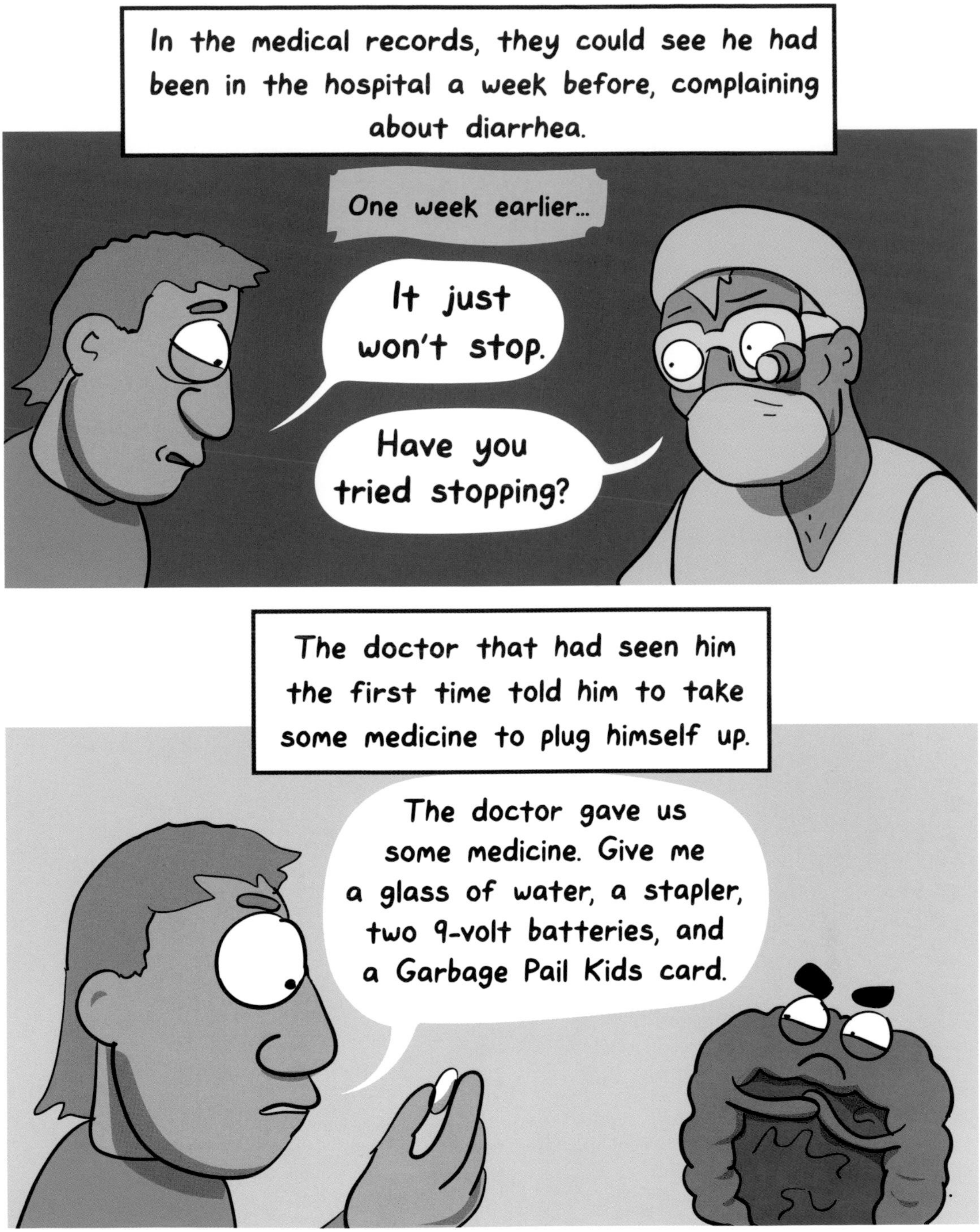
In the medical records, they could see he had been in the hospital a week before, complaining about diarrhea.
One week earlier...
It just won't stop.
Have you tried stopping?
The doctor that had seen him the first time told him to take some medicine to plug himself up.
The doctor gave us some medicine. Give me a glass of water, a stapler, two 9-volt batteries, and a Garbage Pail Kids card.

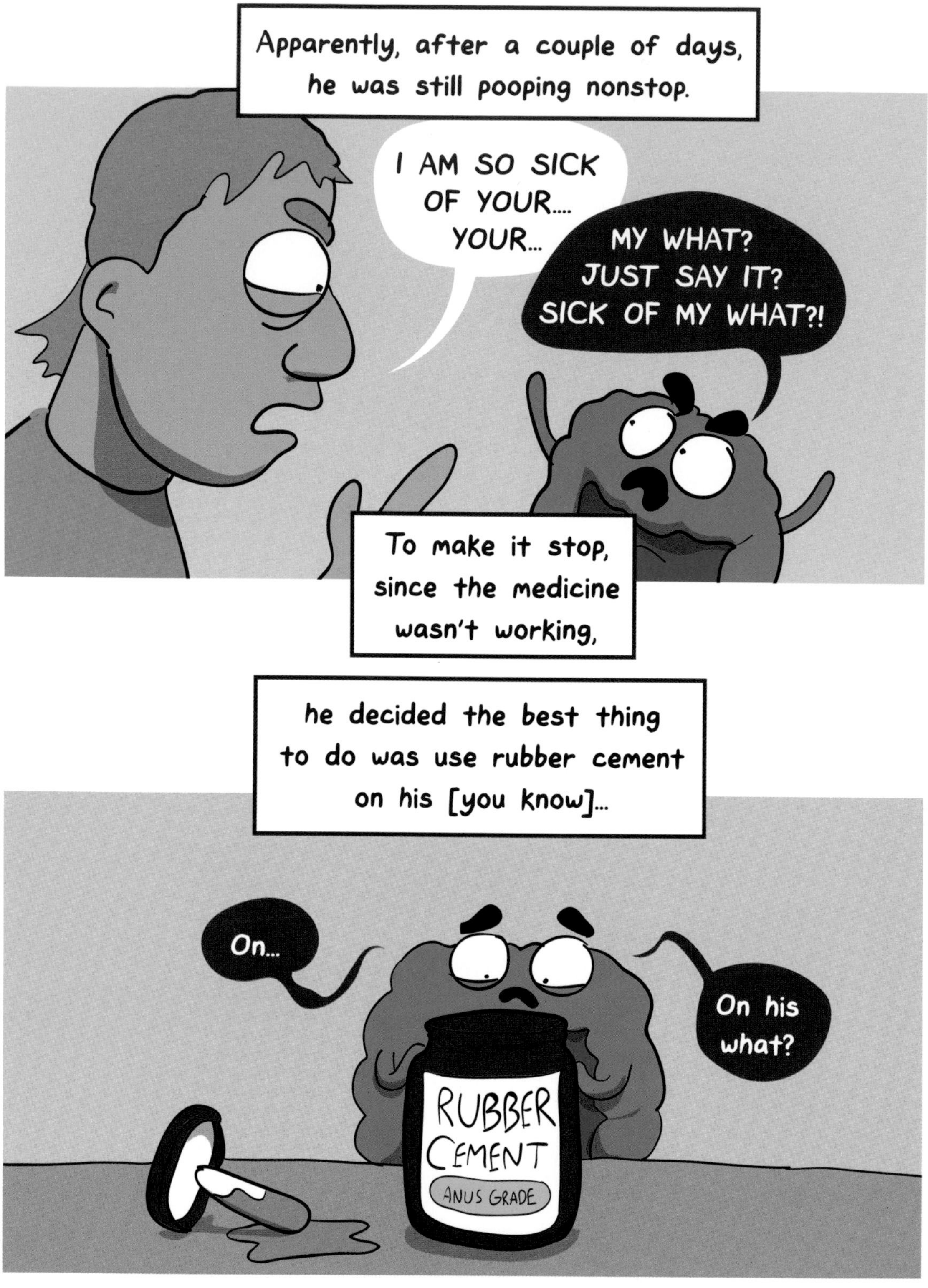
Apparently, after a couple of days, he was still pooping nonstop.
I AM SO SICK OF YOUR.... YOUR...
MY WHAT? JUST SAY IT? SICK OF MY WHAT?!
To make it stop, since the medicine wasn't working,
he decided the best thing to do was use rubber cement on his [you know]...
On...
On his what?
RUBBER CEMENT
ANUS GRADE

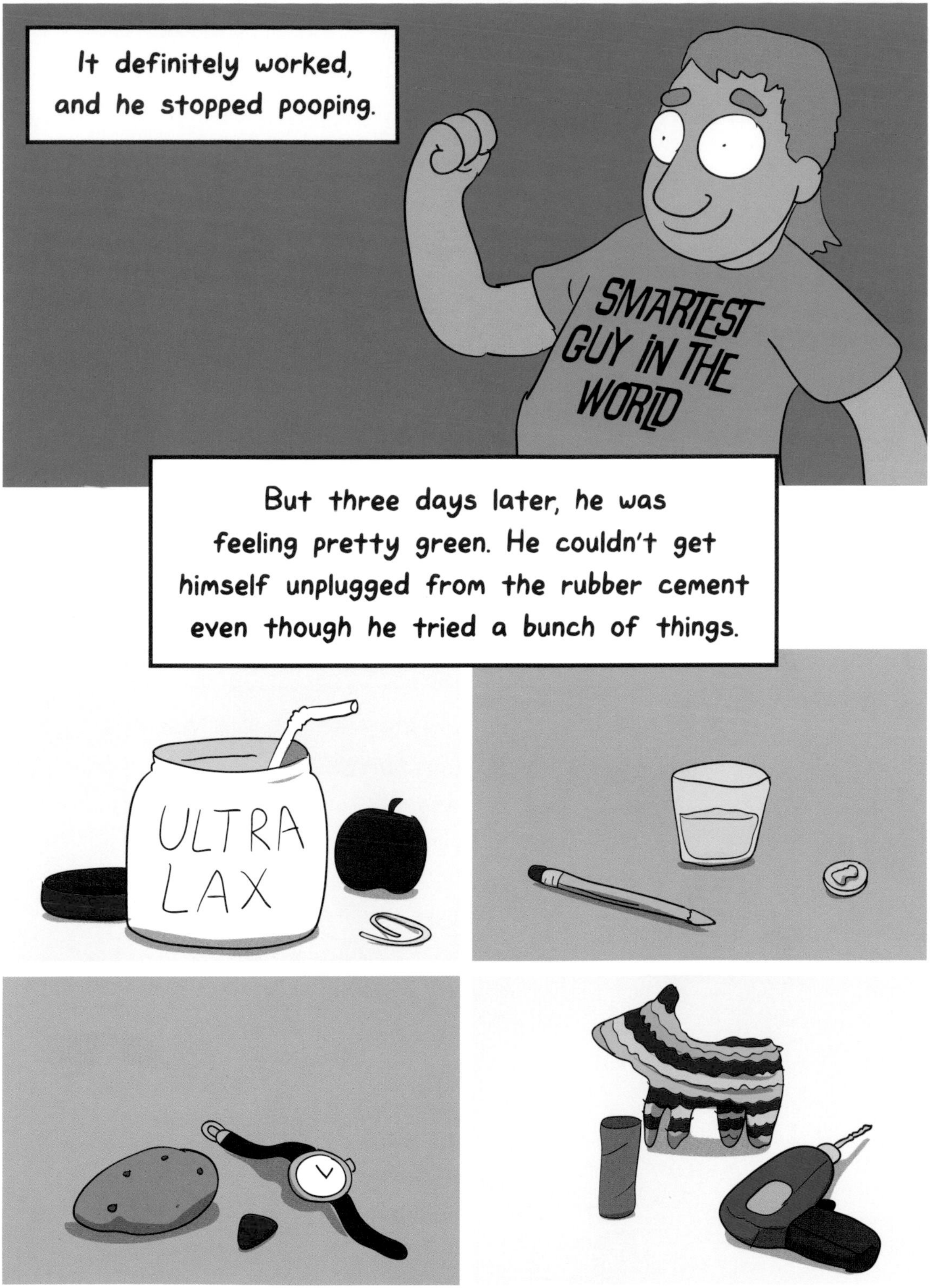
It definitely worked, and he stopped pooping.
SMARTEST GUY IN THE WORLD
But three days later, he was feeling pretty green. He couldn't get himself unplugged from the rubber cement even though he tried a bunch of things.
ULTRA LAX

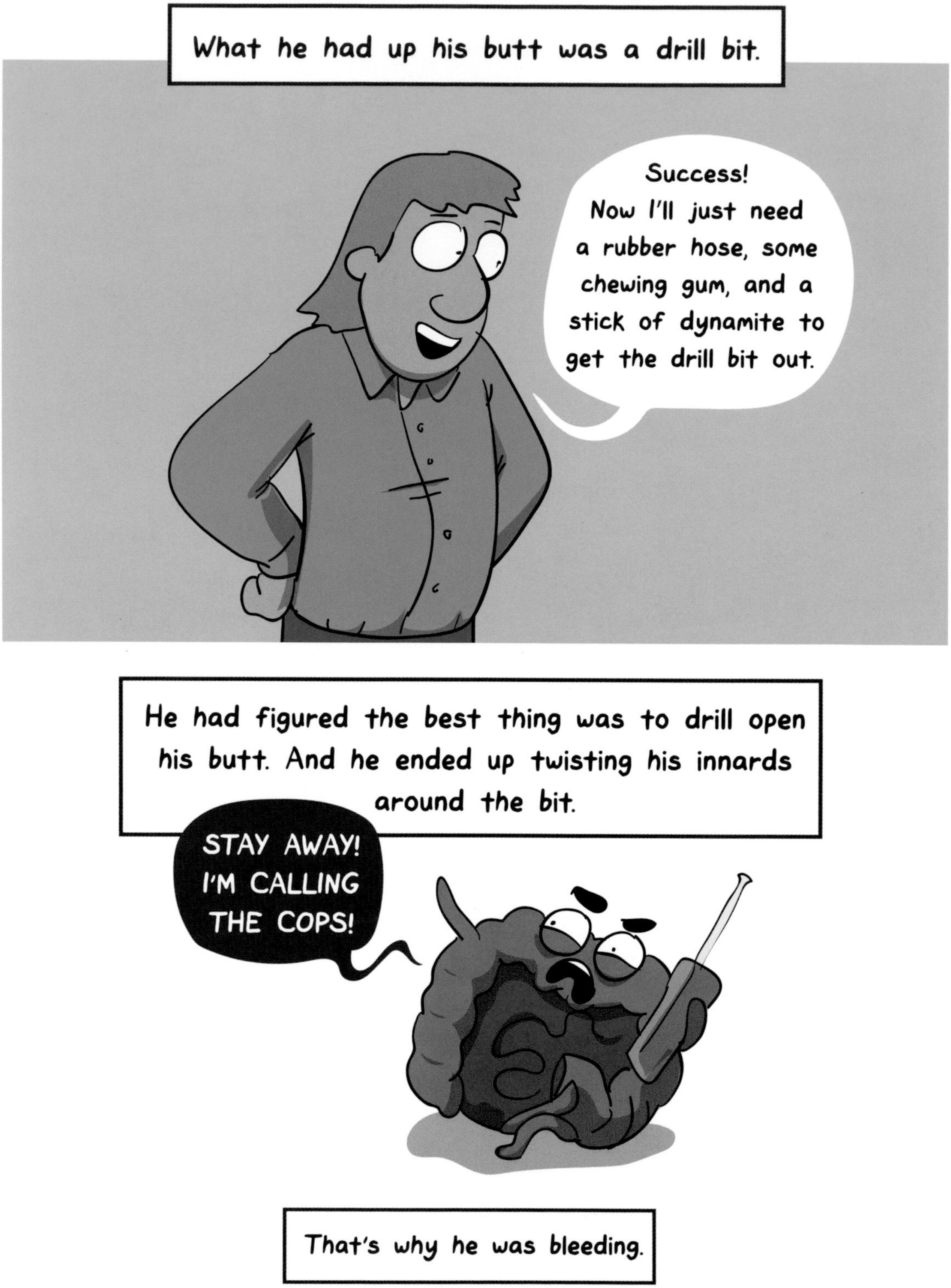
What he had up his butt was a drill bit.
Success! Now I'll just need a rubber hose, some chewing gum, and a stick of dynamite to get the drill bit out.
He had figured the best thing was to drill open his butt. And he ended up twisting his innards around the bit.
STAY AWAY! I'M CALLING THE COPS!
That's why he was bleeding.

Lucky for him, my friend
was a wicked good surgeon.

He survived.

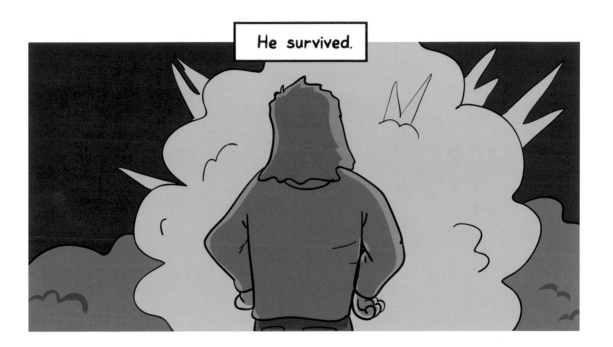

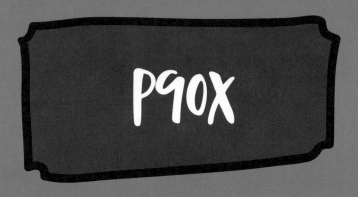

# CHAPTER 16

# P9OX

told by Matt S.

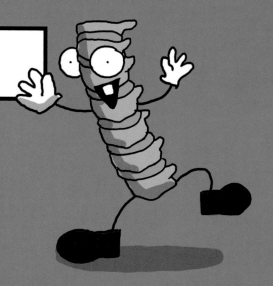

I was working out at my home doing P9OX.

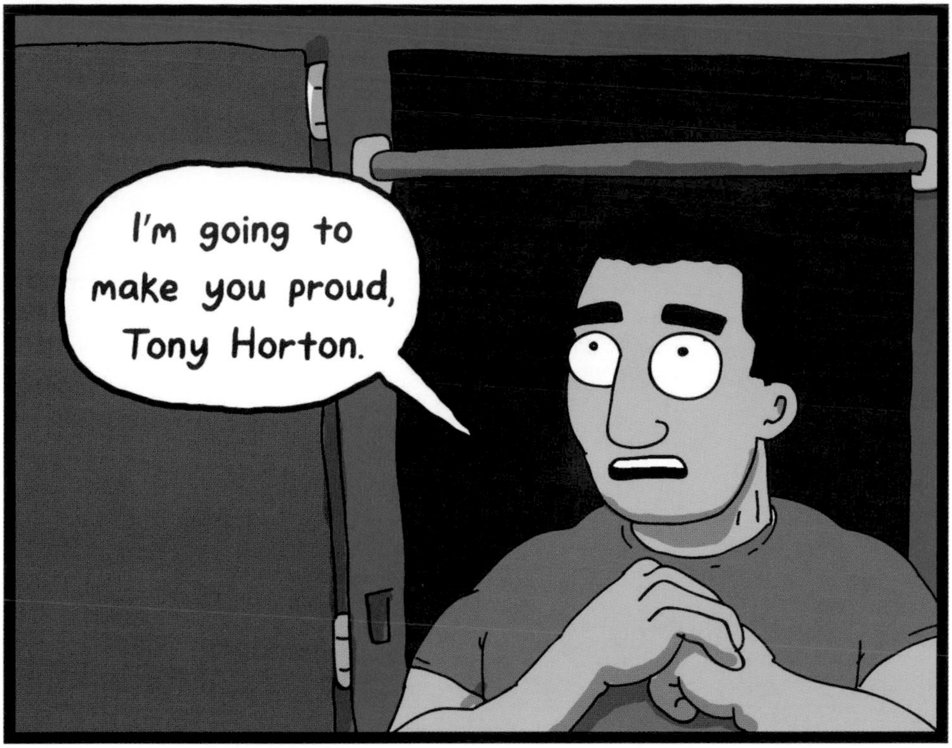
I'm going to make you proud, Tony Horton.

Not really realizing my limitations, I went to do several pull-ups and noticed a sharp pain going down my left arm, starting from my neck.

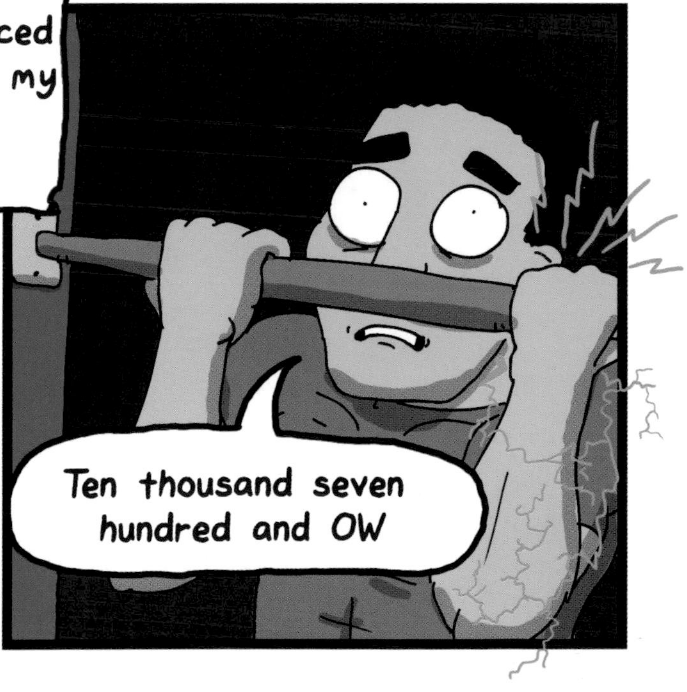
Ten thousand seven hundred and OW

It hurt so much that I couldn't even put a sheet over it.

I tried just about everything to get rid of the pain, including

acupuncture,

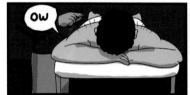

massage,

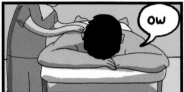

and a chiropractor.

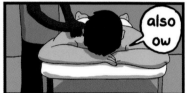

It only made things worse.

So after several weeks of taking Tylenol and ibuprofen, I finally decided to go see the doctor. I got an MRI and the doctor stated that I had a herniated disk in my neck.

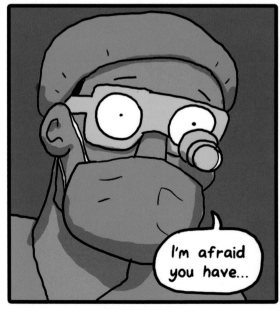

I'm afraid you have...

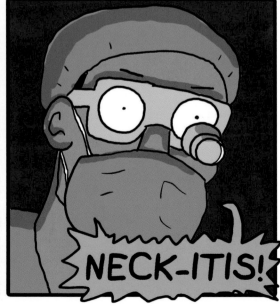

NECK-ITIS!

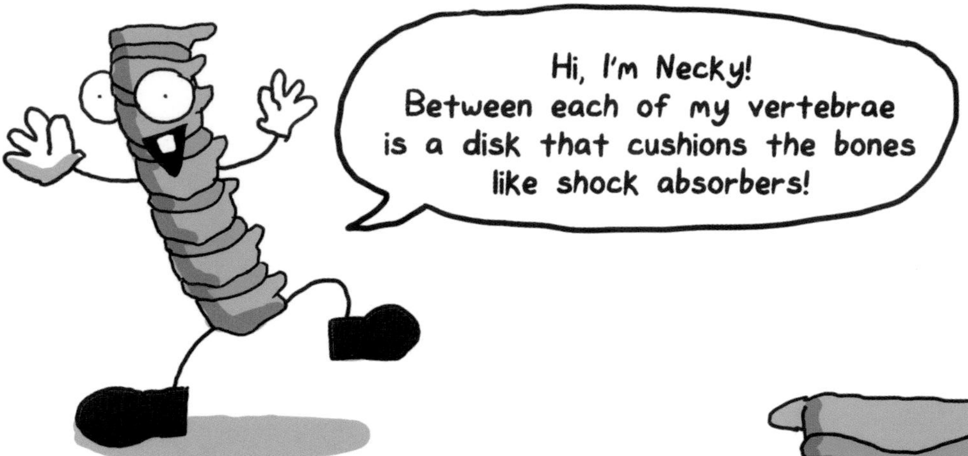
Hi, I'm Necky!
Between each of my vertebrae is a disk that cushions the bones like shock absorbers!

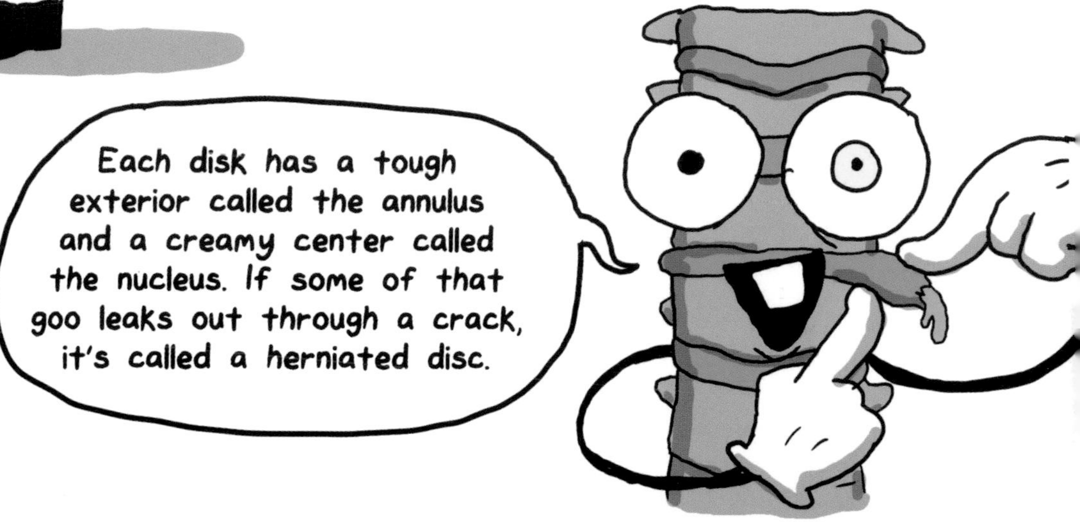
Each disk has a tough exterior called the annulus and a creamy center called the nucleus. If some of that goo leaks out through a crack, it's called a herniated disc.

## Necky's NECK TIPS OF THE DAY:

USE PROPER WEIGHT LIFTING TECHNIQUES
DON'T TURN YOUR HEAD ALL THE WAY AROUND LIKE AN OWL
STRETCH REGULARLY WHEN SITTING FOR A LONG TIME
WEAR A NECK BRACE AS A FASHION STATEMENT
MAINTAIN GOOD POSTURE
NEVER FALL ASLEEP IN A GUILLOTINE
EXERCISE REGULARLY
MINIMIZE BREAK DANCING AT WORK
HEALTHY DIET!

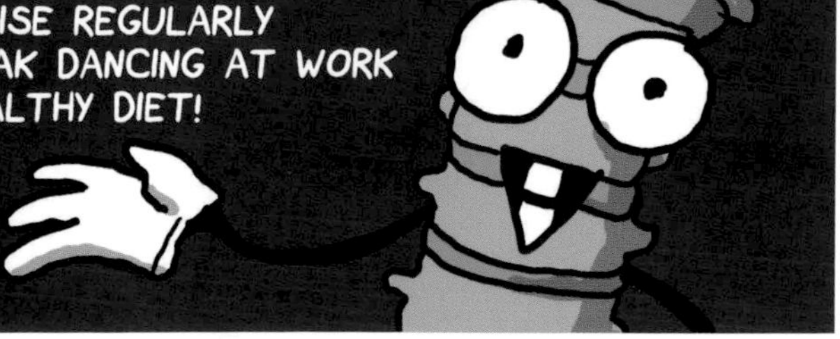

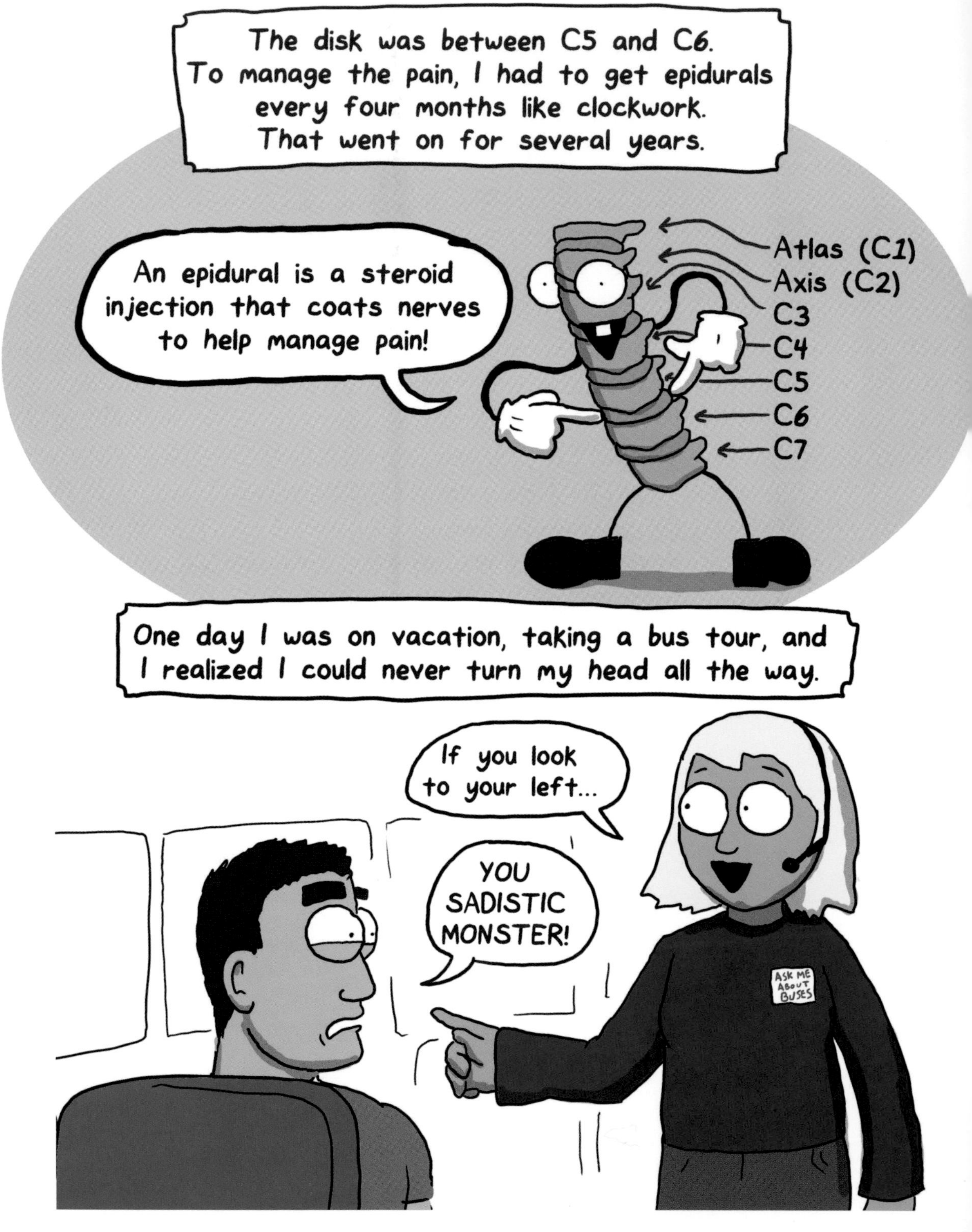
The disk was between C5 and C6. To manage the pain, I had to get epidurals every four months like clockwork. That went on for several years.
An epidural is a steroid injection that coats nerves to help manage pain!
Atlas (C1)
Axis (C2)
C3
C4
C5
C6
C7
One day I was on vacation, taking a bus tour, and I realized I could never turn my head all the way.
If you look to your left...
YOU SADISTIC MONSTER!
ASK ME ABOUT BUSES

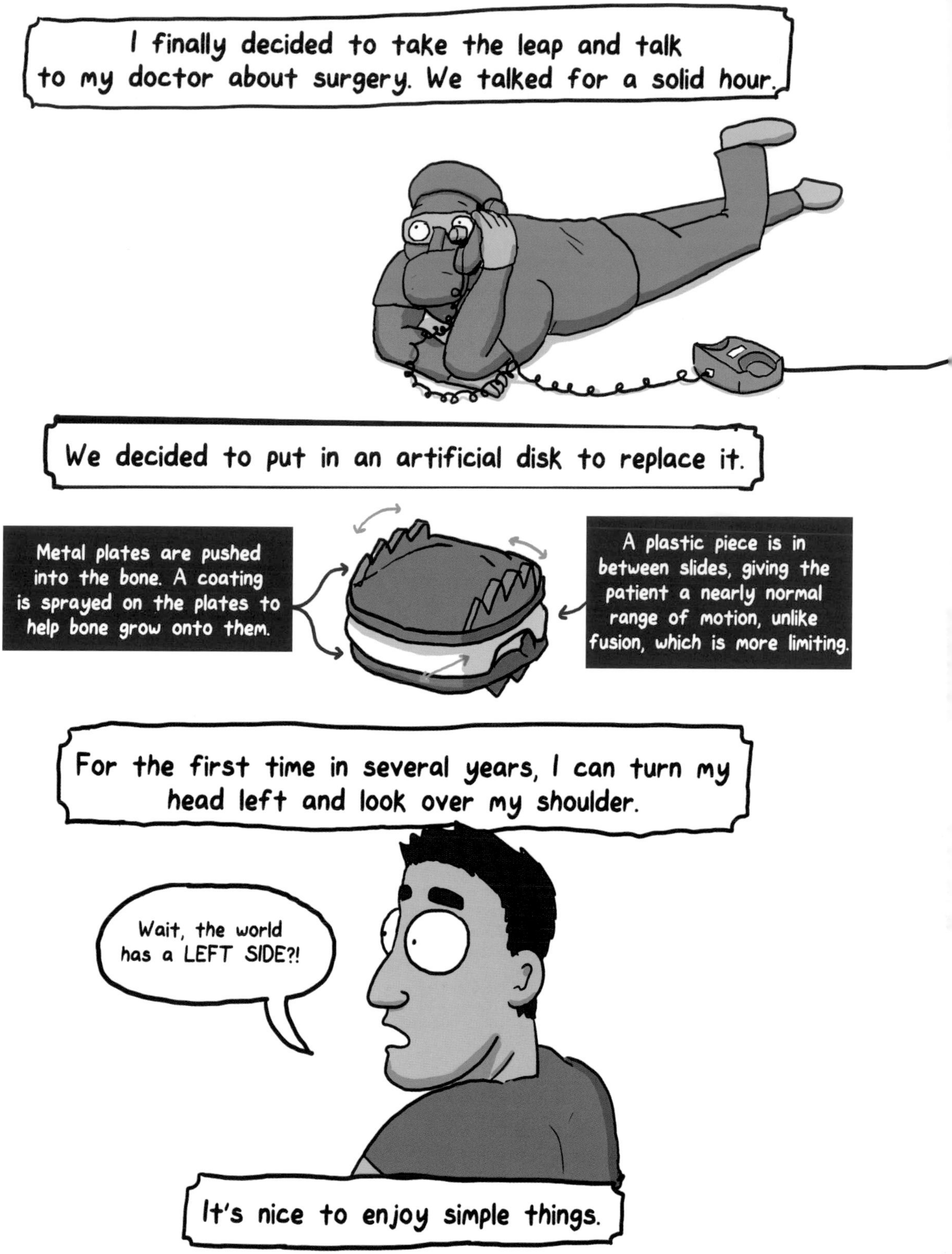
I finally decided to take the leap and talk to my doctor about surgery. We talked for a solid hour.
We decided to put in an artificial disk to replace it.
Metal plates are pushed into the bone. A coating is sprayed on the plates to help bone grow onto them.
A plastic piece is in between slides, giving the patient a nearly normal range of motion, unlike fusion, which is more limiting.
For the first time in several years, I can turn my head left and look over my shoulder.
Wait, the world has a LEFT SIDE?!
It's nice to enjoy simple things.

# CHAPTER 17

# ATTACK of THE SPINE

## told by El

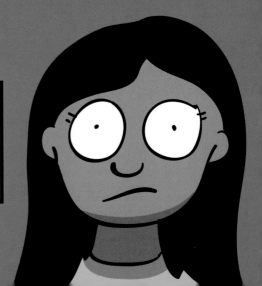

I have a long, raised scar down my side, across my tummy, and down again. When folks see it and say,

"Oh! Were you bitten by a shark?"
I can just reply with,
"Nah, but surgeons broke my spine in nine places."

What actually happened is my spine tried to kill me (twice).
BWA HA HA HA cough HACK

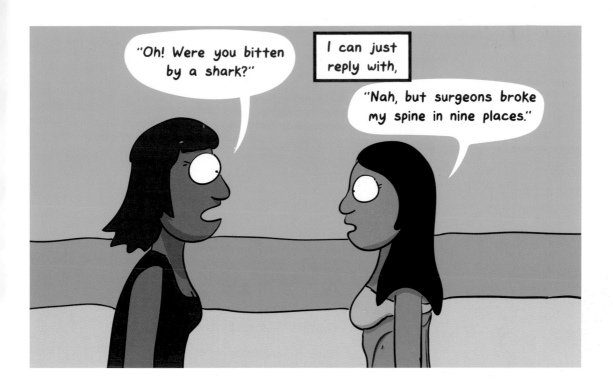

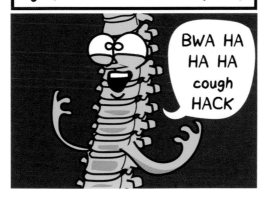

When I was a kid, I had scoliosis.
A sideways curve in the spine, it's pretty common.
Except I had *double* scoliosis,

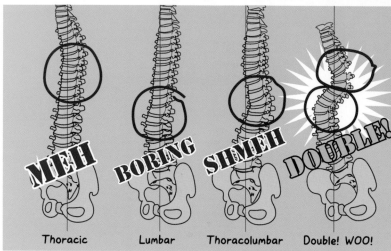

MEH

BORING

SHMEH

DOUBLE!

Thoracic    Lumbar    Thoracolumbar    Double! WOO!

Scoliosis is defined as a sideways curve in the spine and varies in intensity.

A curve usually goes in a C or backwards-C shape, but sometimes will do a double curve like the letter S.

Treatment varies depending on the severity.

which sounds hilarious,
but it is horrifying.

Instead of being extremely curved to one side,
my spine concertinaed back on itself,

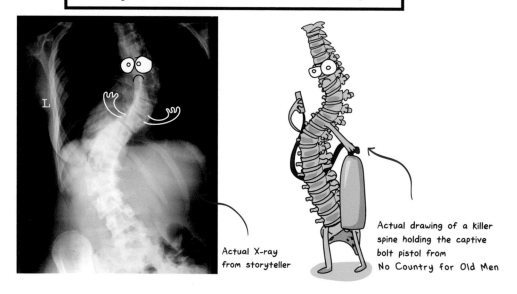

L

Actual X-ray
from storyteller

Actual drawing of a killer spine holding the captive bolt pistol from
No Country for Old Men

Wood it hewp if I maked sumpin'?
Give it a rest, Gallbladder!

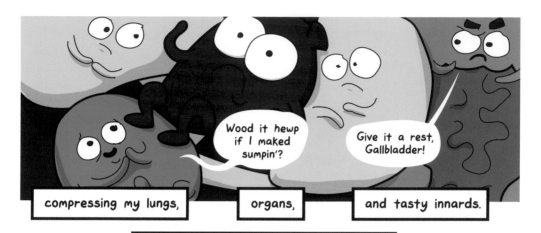

compressing my lungs,

organs,

and tasty innards.

By the time I was 12, I had space for only one-third of my left lung.

HELP HEEEEEELLLLP!
SPINE CRUSH! HADOUKEN!
Are you going to be wheezing all night, or what's the deal?

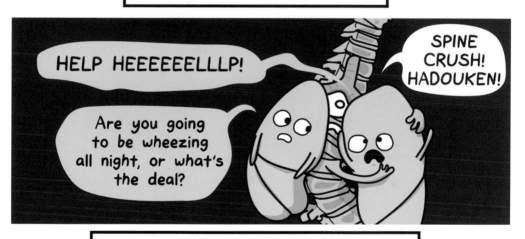

I was going to die at some point if it continued.

(Twelve-year-old me did not know this.)

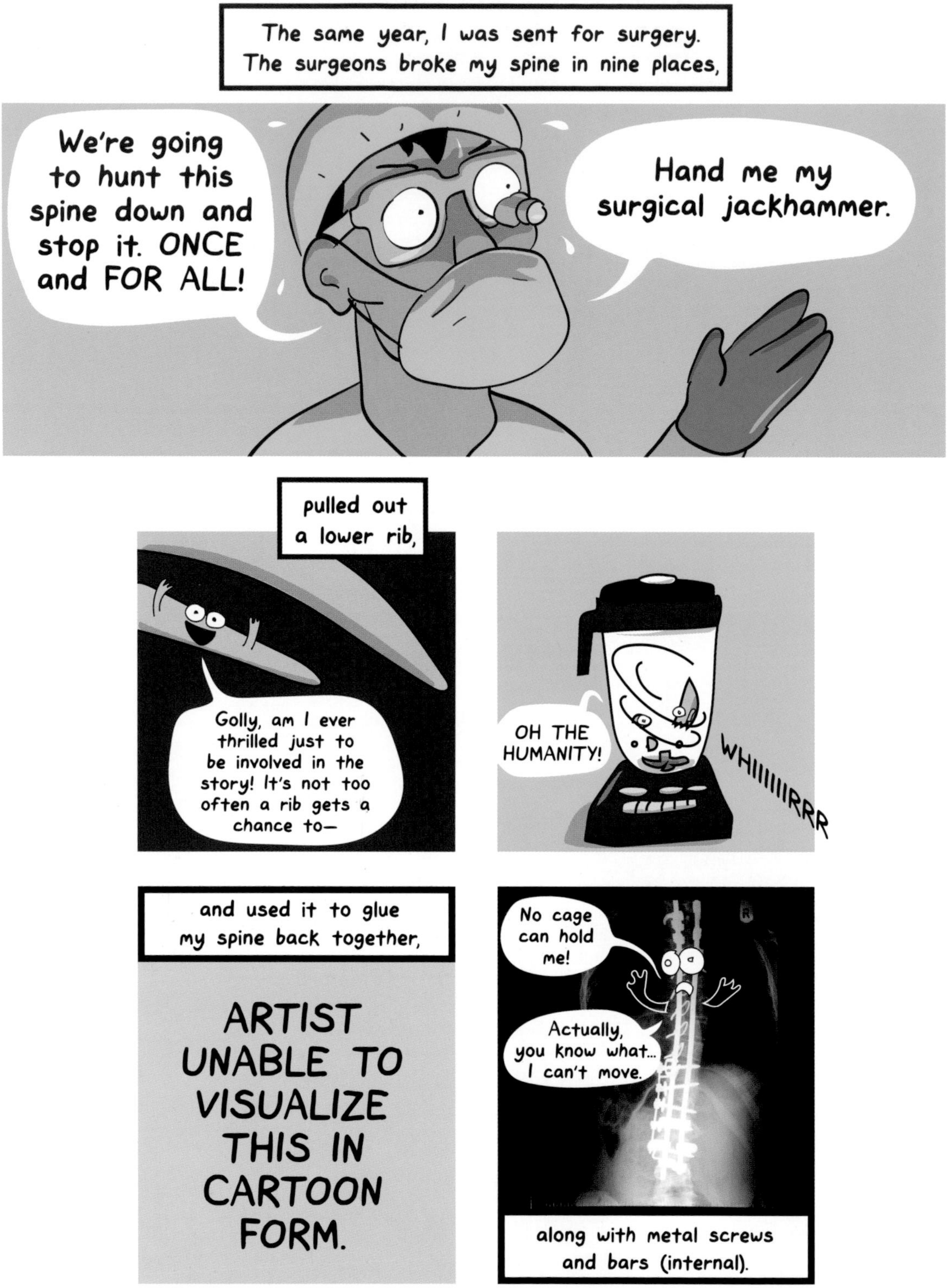

The same year, I was sent for surgery. The surgeons broke my spine in nine places,
We're going to hunt this spine down and stop it. ONCE and FOR ALL!
Hand me my surgical jackhammer.
pulled out a lower rib,
Golly, am I ever thrilled just to be involved in the story! It's not too often a rib gets a chance to—
OH THE HUMANITY!
WHIIIIIIRRR
and used it to glue my spine back together,
ARTIST UNABLE TO VISUALIZE THIS IN CARTOON FORM.
No cage can hold me!
Actually, you know what... I can't move.
along with metal screws and bars (internal).

I also grew over two inches taller.

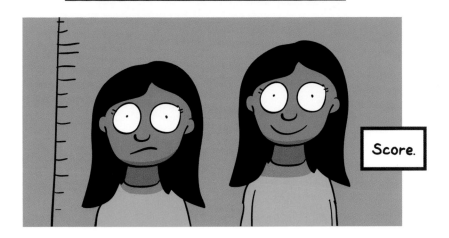

Score.

The metalwork for this kind of surgery stays inside the patient, unlike when you break a hand or wrist, because nobody wants to cut you open and get them back.

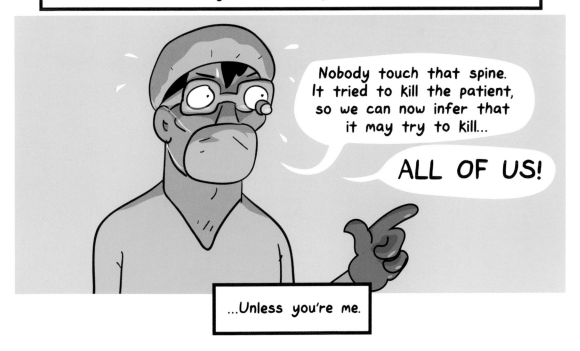

Nobody touch that spine. It tried to kill the patient, so we can now infer that it may try to kill...

ALL OF US!

...Unless you're me.

At age 18, I started to get cranky all the time, hated everything, and didn't care about my exams, or much else.

Whatever.
What EVER.

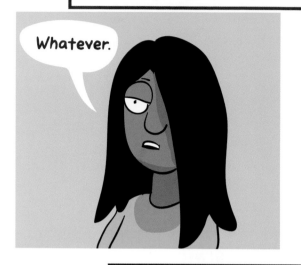

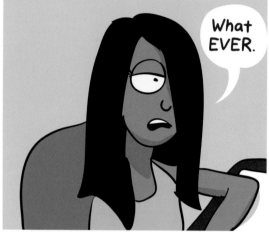

Eventually, the doctors found that instead of being a petulant little mardy-arse teenager, I was actually dying from internal infection.

The metal had become infected and formed an antibiotic-resistant biofilm around itself.

We are spine.
We are one.

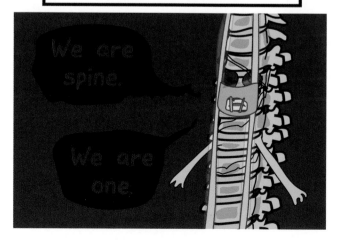

The only answer was to get it out again, this time for good. I remember getting the news that I had to go through another massive spinal surgery and being more interested in getting a cookie from the hospital store,

Whatever.

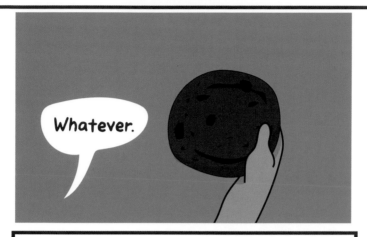

and that the copy of National Geographic had a cute fox on the cover.

NATIONAL
Whatever.

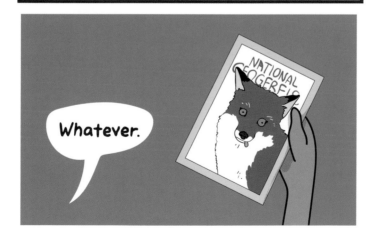

That's how apathetic and disconnected I was at that point.

The metalwork came out of surgery before I did,

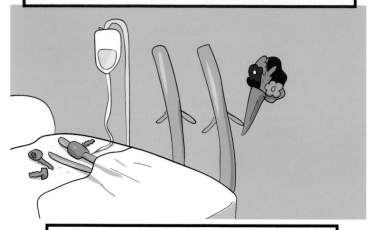

and was handed to my parents in a damp, clear plastic bag. It was not as clean as they'd hoped it would be.

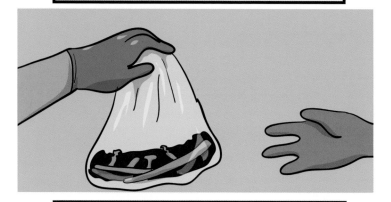

I have it in a box under my desk these days. Someday, I'm going to see if I can convince a jeweler to do something with it.

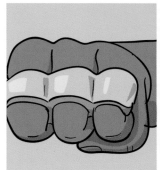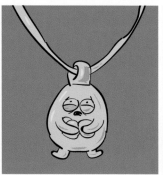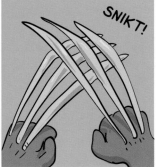

SNIKT!

It's been 10 years and my spine has not made another threat on my life thus far.

I just don't understand...
All I ever wanted to do was squish all the organs and gain their powers!
Is that so weird?
Actual X-ray from after the second surgery*
*Spine dialogue paraphrased

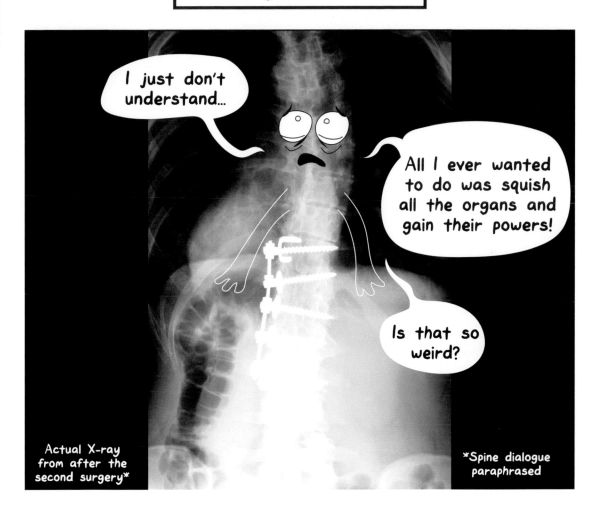

# CHAPTER 18

# BABY'S FIRST DENTAL EMERGENCY

## told by A. Mohamad

I'm a dentist,
and one day the following
saga unfolded in our clinic.

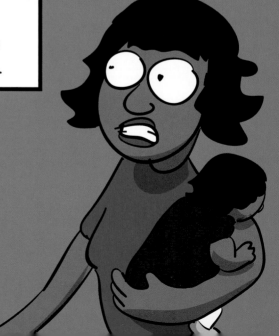

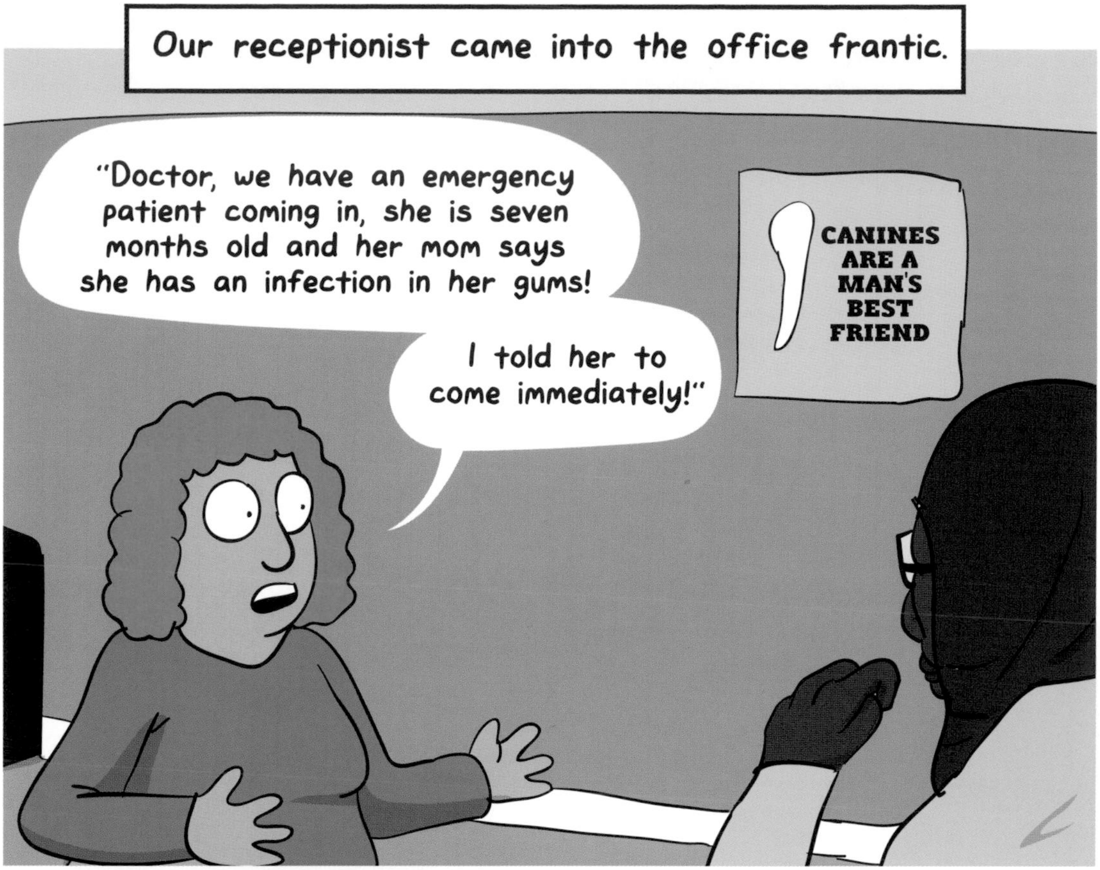
Our receptionist came into the office frantic.
"Doctor, we have an emergency patient coming in, she is seven months old and her mom says she has an infection in her gums!
I told her to come immediately!"
CANINES ARE A MAN'S BEST FRIEND

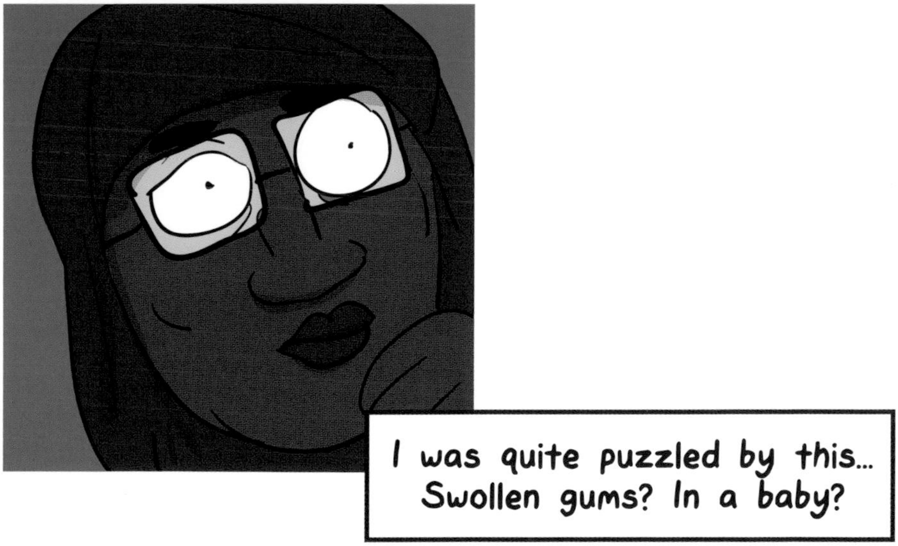
I was quite puzzled by this... Swollen gums? In a baby?

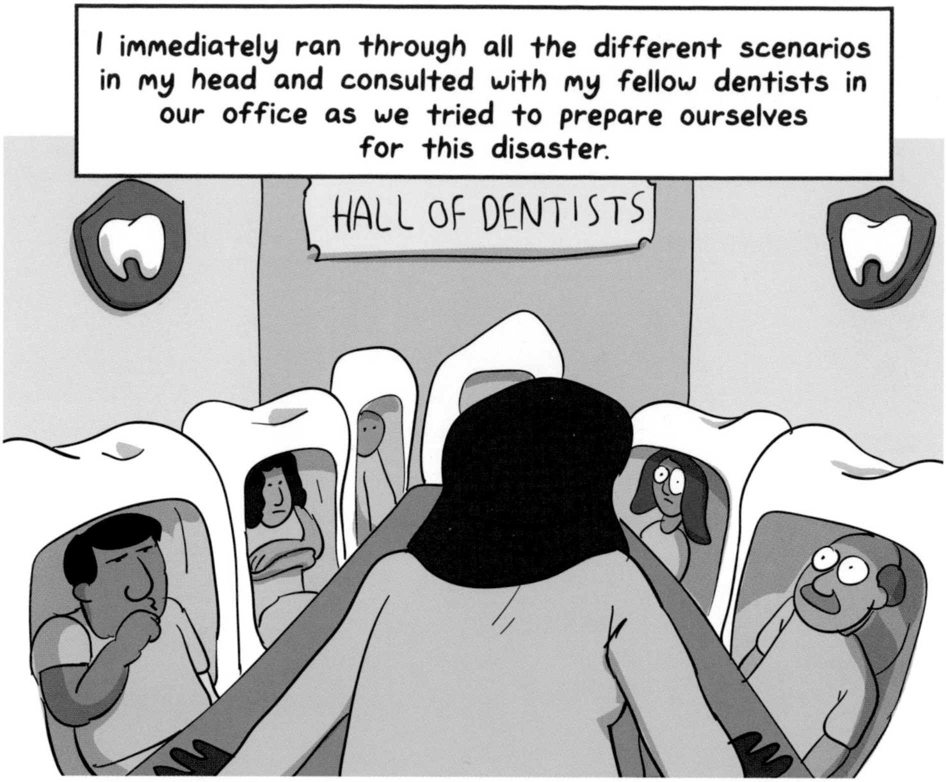
I immediately ran through all the different scenarios in my head and consulted with my fellow dentists in our office as we tried to prepare ourselves for this disaster.
HALL OF DENTISTS

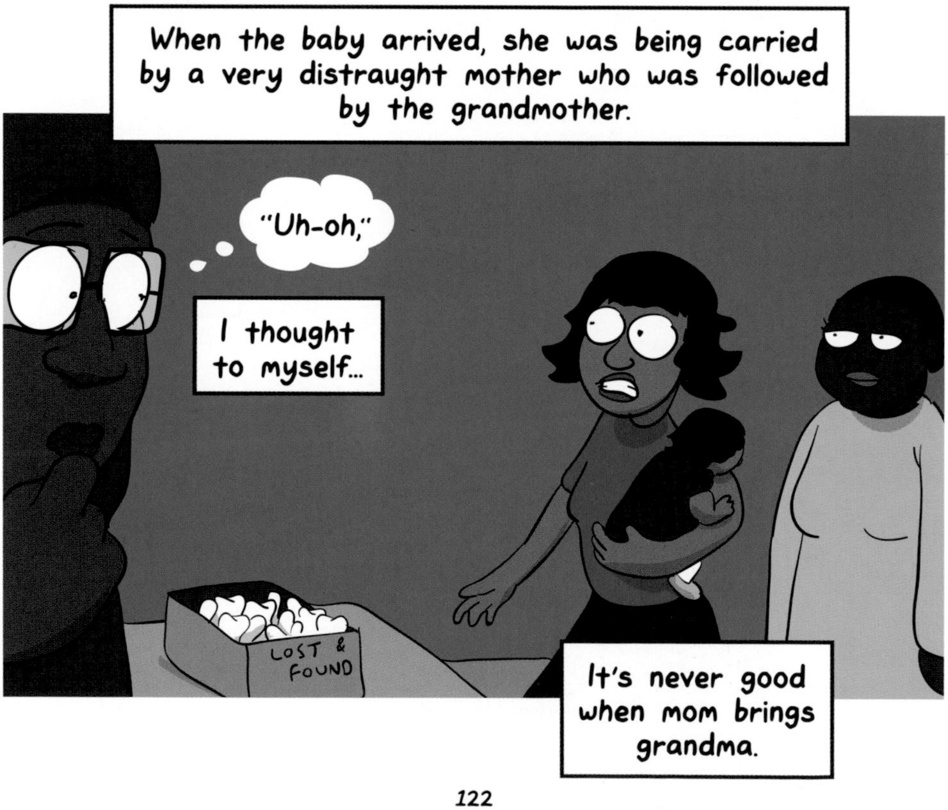
When the baby arrived, she was being carried by a very distraught mother who was followed by the grandmother.
"Uh-oh,"
I thought to myself...
LOST & FOUND
It's never good when mom brings grandma.

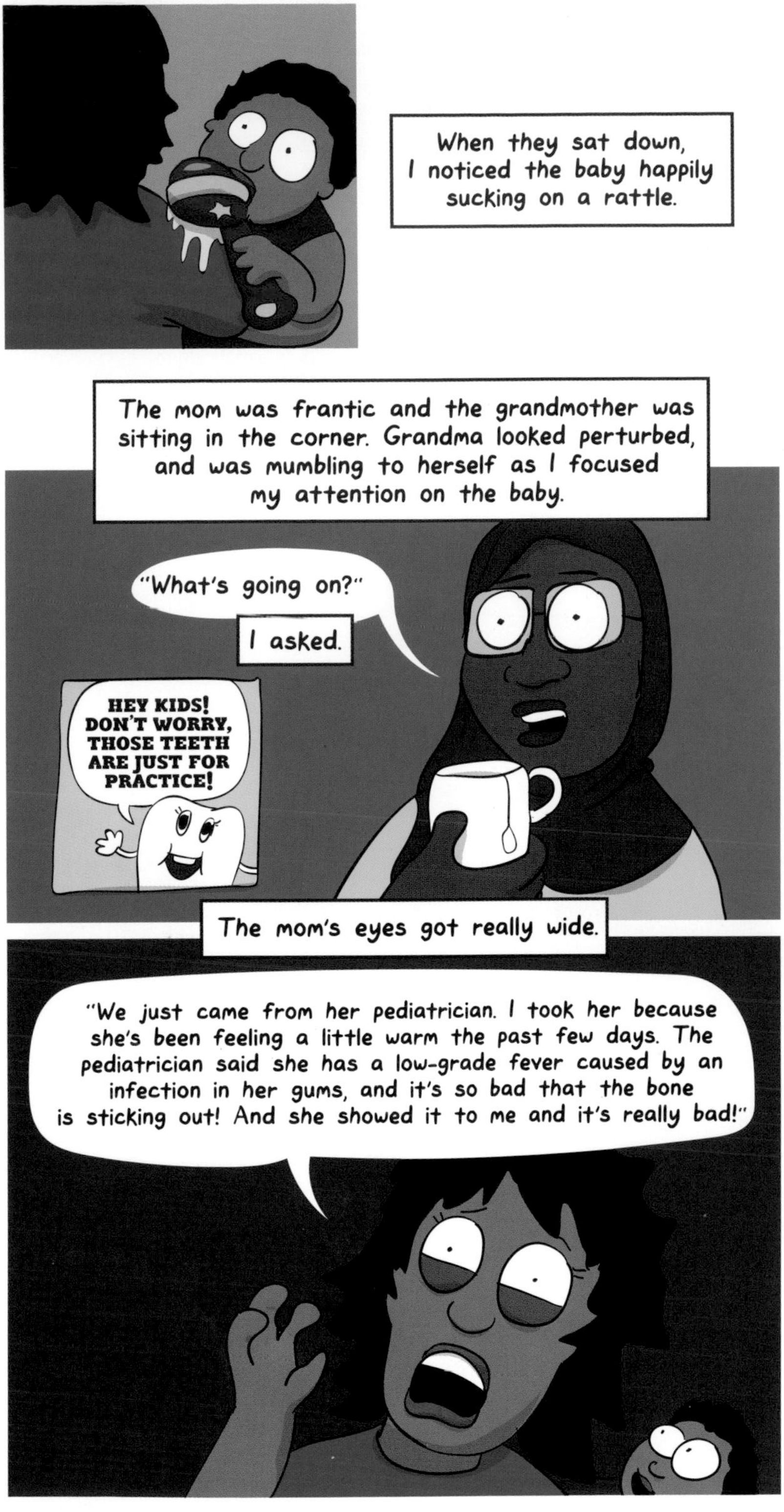
When they sat down, I noticed the baby happily sucking on a rattle.
The mom was frantic and the grandmother was sitting in the corner. Grandma looked perturbed, and was mumbling to herself as I focused my attention on the baby.
"What's going on?"
I asked.
HEY KIDS! DON'T WORRY, THOSE TEETH ARE JUST FOR PRACTICE!
The mom's eyes got really wide.
"We just came from her pediatrician. I took her because she's been feeling a little warm the past few days. The pediatrician said she has a low-grade fever caused by an infection in her gums, and it's so bad that the bone is sticking out! And she showed it to me and it's really bad!"

This was news to me...
I opened my mouth to speak but
grandma interjected,

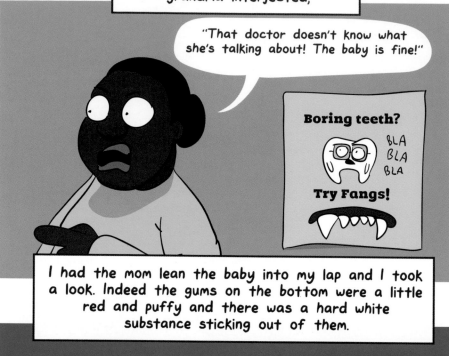

"That doctor doesn't know what
she's talking about! The baby is fine!"

**Boring teeth?**

BLA
BLA
BLA

**Try Fangs!**

I had the mom lean the baby into my lap and I took a look. Indeed the gums on the bottom were a little red and puffy and there was a hard white substance sticking out of them.

I looked up at the mom
and grinned,

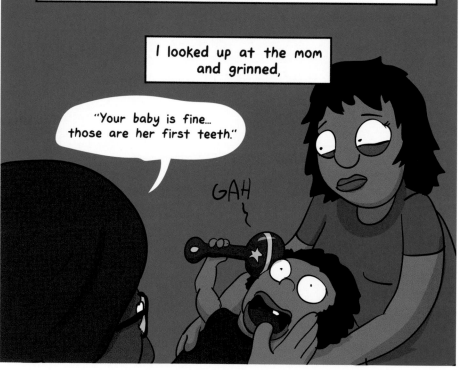

"Your baby is fine...
those are her first teeth."

GAH

Grandma stood up:

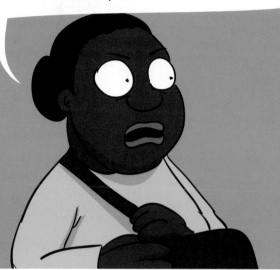

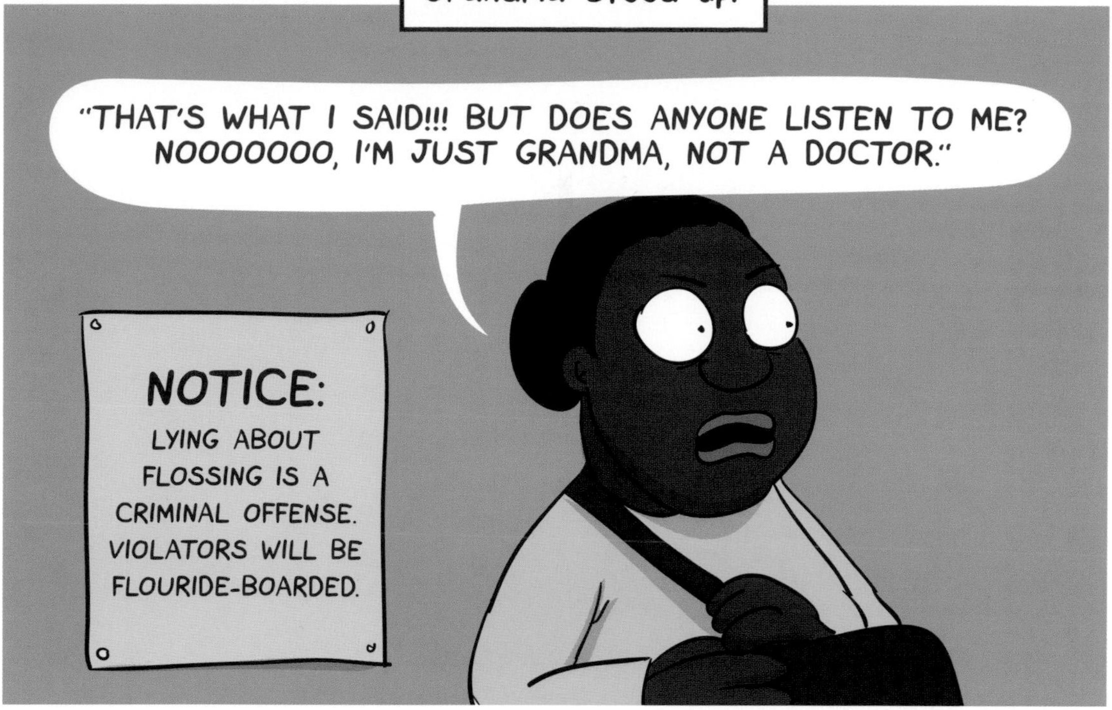

"THAT'S WHAT I SAID!!! BUT DOES ANYONE LISTEN TO ME? NOOOOOOO, I'M JUST GRANDMA, NOT A DOCTOR."

NOTICE:

LYING ABOUT FLOSSING IS A CRIMINAL OFFENSE. VIOLATORS WILL BE FLOURIDE-BOARDED.

After that, I told the mom that she should listen to her own mother, we all had a good chuckle, and the baby got a sticker.

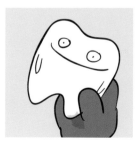

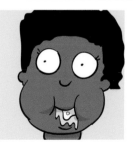

Now you think it would end there, right?

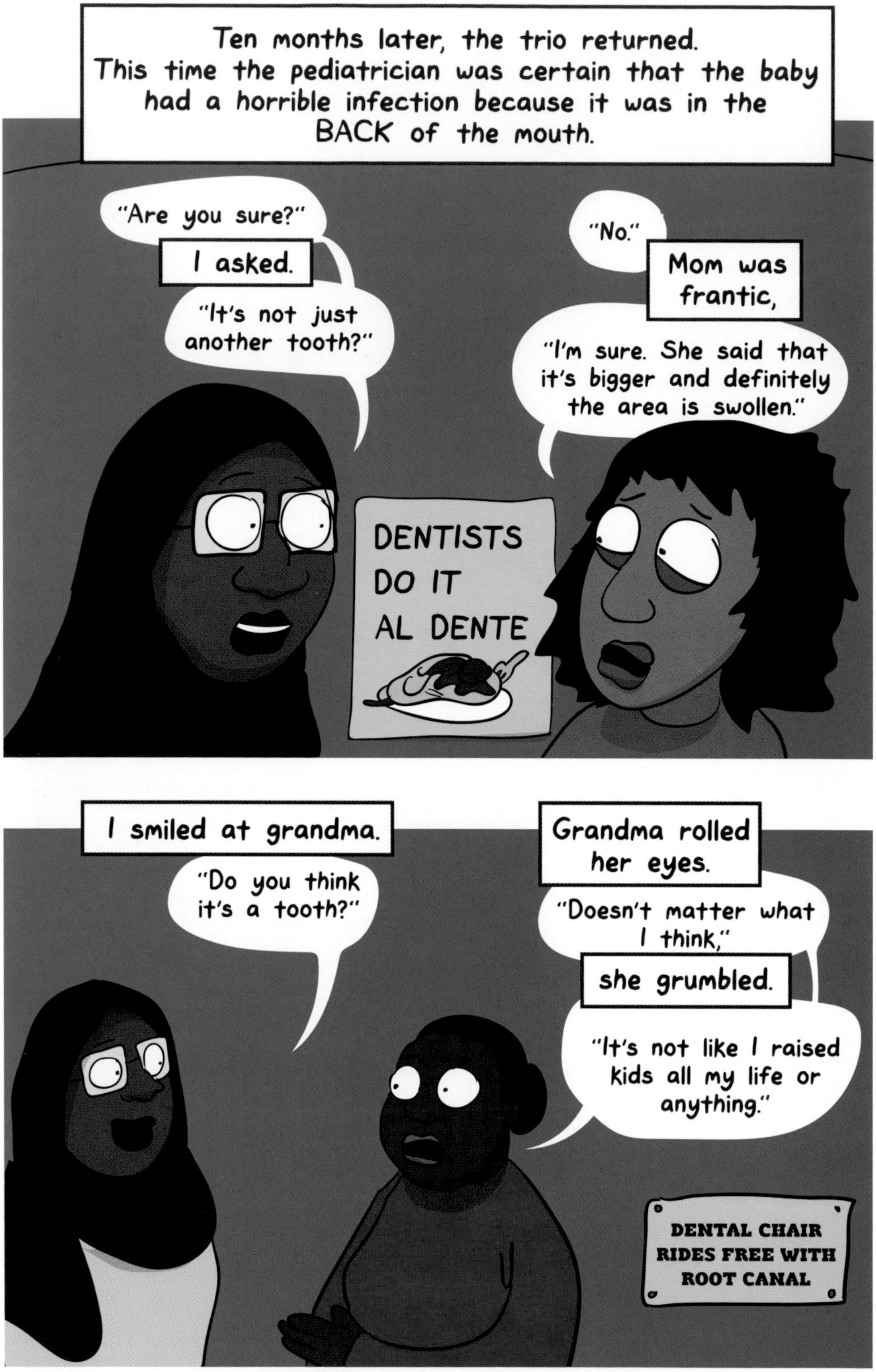

Ten months later, the trio returned. This time the pediatrician was certain that the baby had a horrible infection because it was in the BACK of the mouth.
"Are you sure?"
I asked.
"It's not just another tooth?"
"No."
Mom was frantic,
"I'm sure. She said that it's bigger and definitely the area is swollen."
DENTISTS DO IT AL DENTE
I smiled at grandma.
"Do you think it's a tooth?"
Grandma rolled her eyes.
"Doesn't matter what I think,"
she grumbled.
"It's not like I raised kids all my life or anything."
DENTAL CHAIR RIDES FREE WITH ROOT CANAL

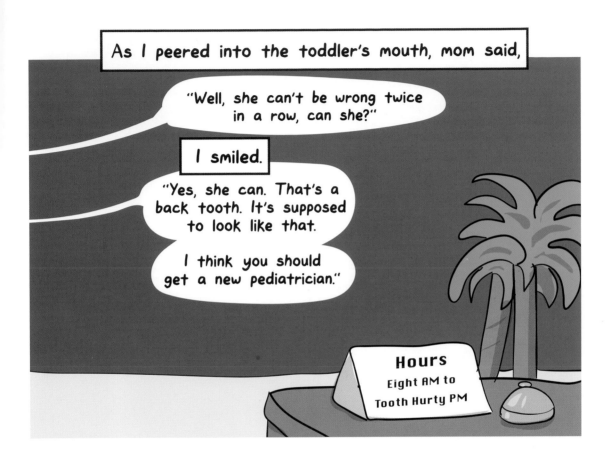

As I peered into the toddler's mouth, mom said,

"Well, she can't be wrong twice in a row, can she?"

I smiled.

"Yes, she can. That's a back tooth. It's supposed to look like that.

I think you should get a new pediatrician."

Hours
Eight AM to
Tooth Hurty PM

tooth →

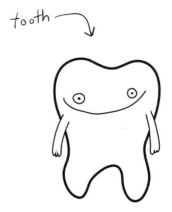

# CHAPTER 19

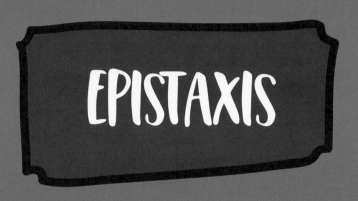

## EPISTAXIS

told by Eli

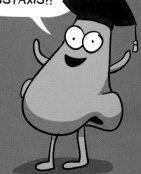

Hey there, kids! I'm NOSEY the NOSE! Did you know that the technical term for a nosebleed is EPISTAXIS?!

I used to have nosebleeds that were so bad the blood would start to travel up to my eyes,

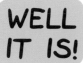

WELL IT IS!

and I would bleed through my eyes and my nose at the same time.

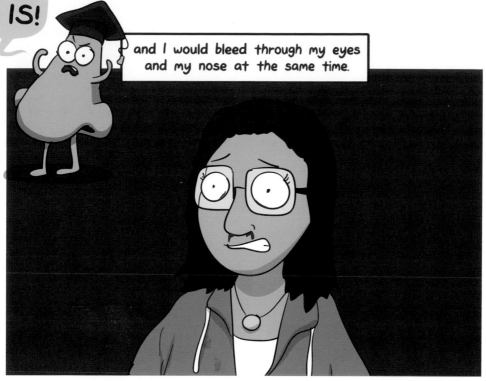

It looked like I was dying of a rare disease, but even so, I thought it was pretty cool to cry blood.

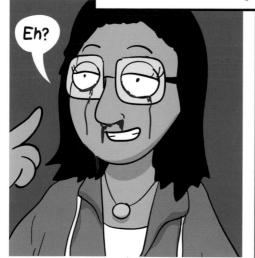

Eh?

A bad nosebleed can back up through the nasolacrimal duct into the eye! That's the same duct that normally DRAINS tears from your eye! EYE CAN'T BE-L-EYE-V IT!

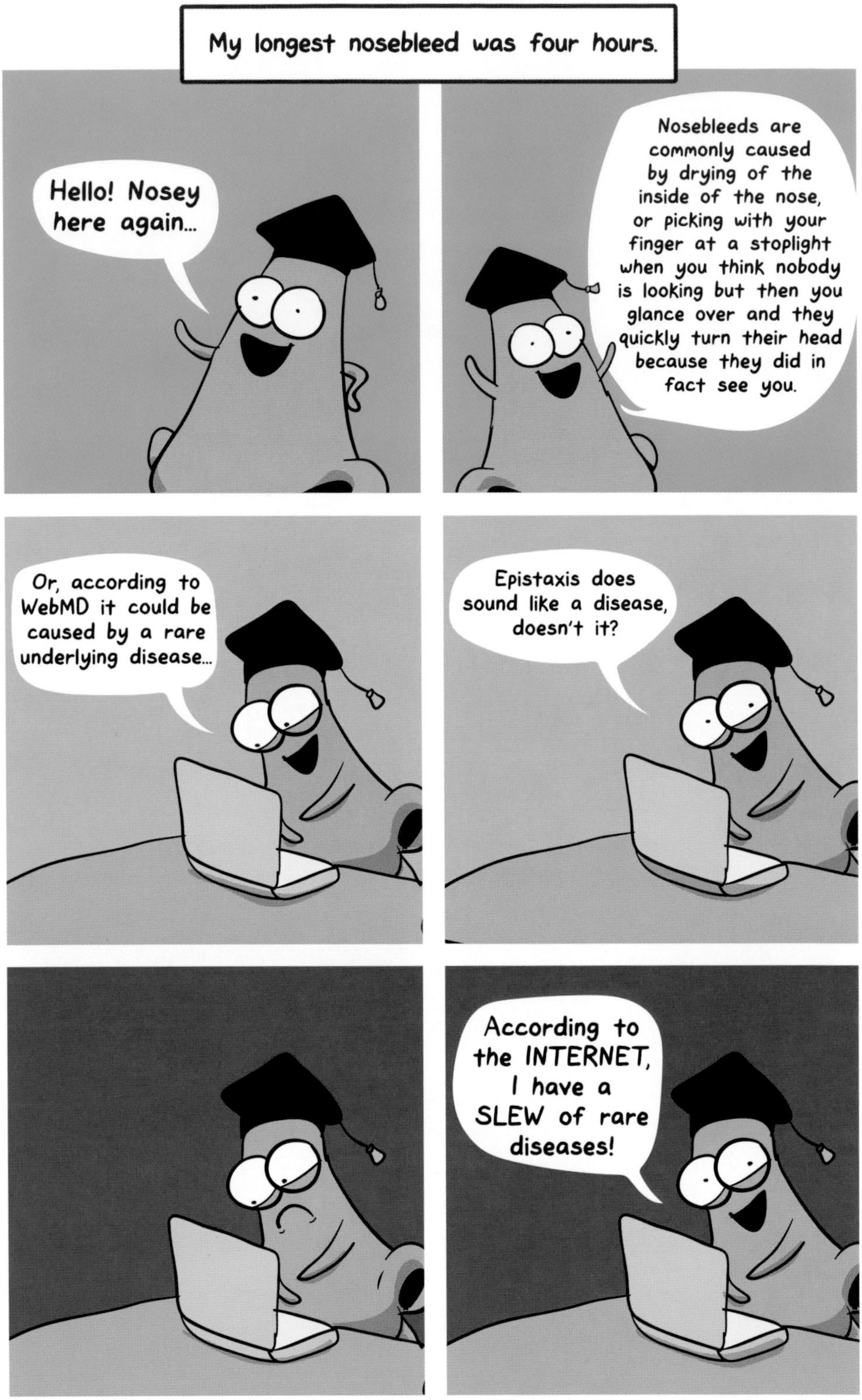
My longest nosebleed was four hours.
Hello! Nosey here again...
Nosebleeds are commonly caused by drying of the inside of the nose, or picking with your finger at a stoplight when you think nobody is looking but then you glance over and they quickly turn their head because they did in fact see you.
Or, according to WebMD it could be caused by a rare underlying disease...
Epistaxis does sound like a disease, doesn't it?
According to the INTERNET, I have a SLEW of rare diseases!

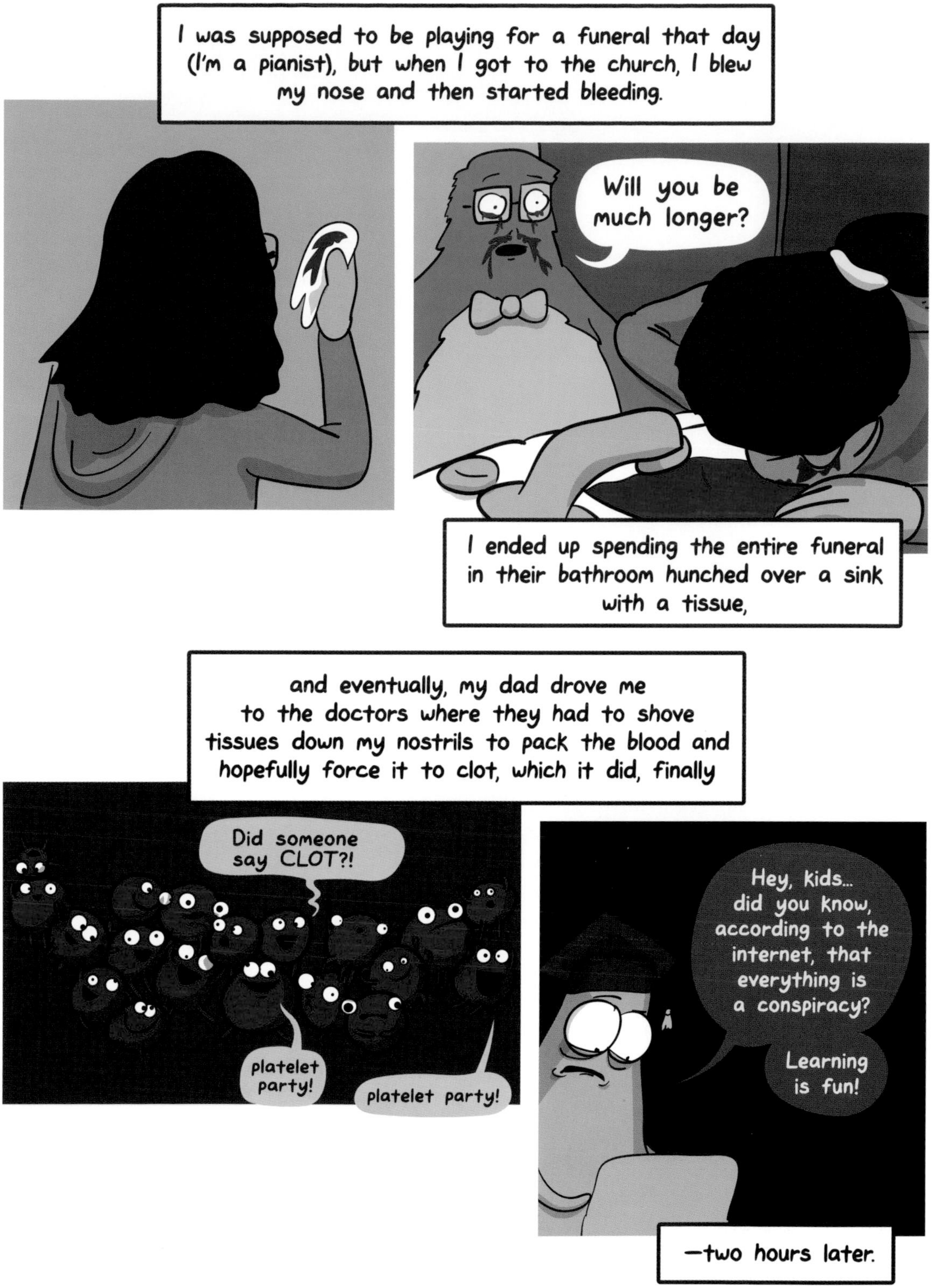
I was supposed to be playing for a funeral that day (I'm a pianist), but when I got to the church, I blew my nose and then started bleeding.
Will you be much longer?
I ended up spending the entire funeral in their bathroom hunched over a sink with a tissue,
and eventually, my dad drove me to the doctors where they had to shove tissues down my nostrils to pack the blood and hopefully force it to clot, which it did, finally
Did someone say CLOT?!
platelet party!
platelet party!
Hey, kids... did you know, according to the internet, that everything is a conspiracy?
Learning is fun!
—two hours later.

By that point in time, my nose was so full of blood clots I couldn't breathe through it for a day.

I think we may have overdone it.
Don't be such an anticoagulant!
platelet party!
platelet party!
platelet party!

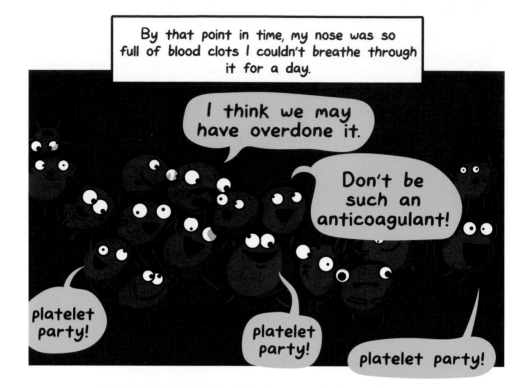

The nosebleeds ended up happening so bad and were so often, I went to an ENT to have my nose assessed, and I was told I had enlarged veins in my left nostril, which were very thin, and that was causing the issue.

I'm afraid you suffer from... RECURRENT ANTERIOR EPISTAXIS!
You mean frequent nosebleeds?
How should I know?
ENT

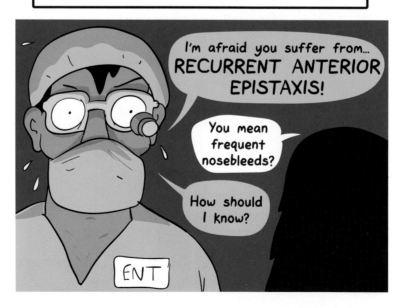

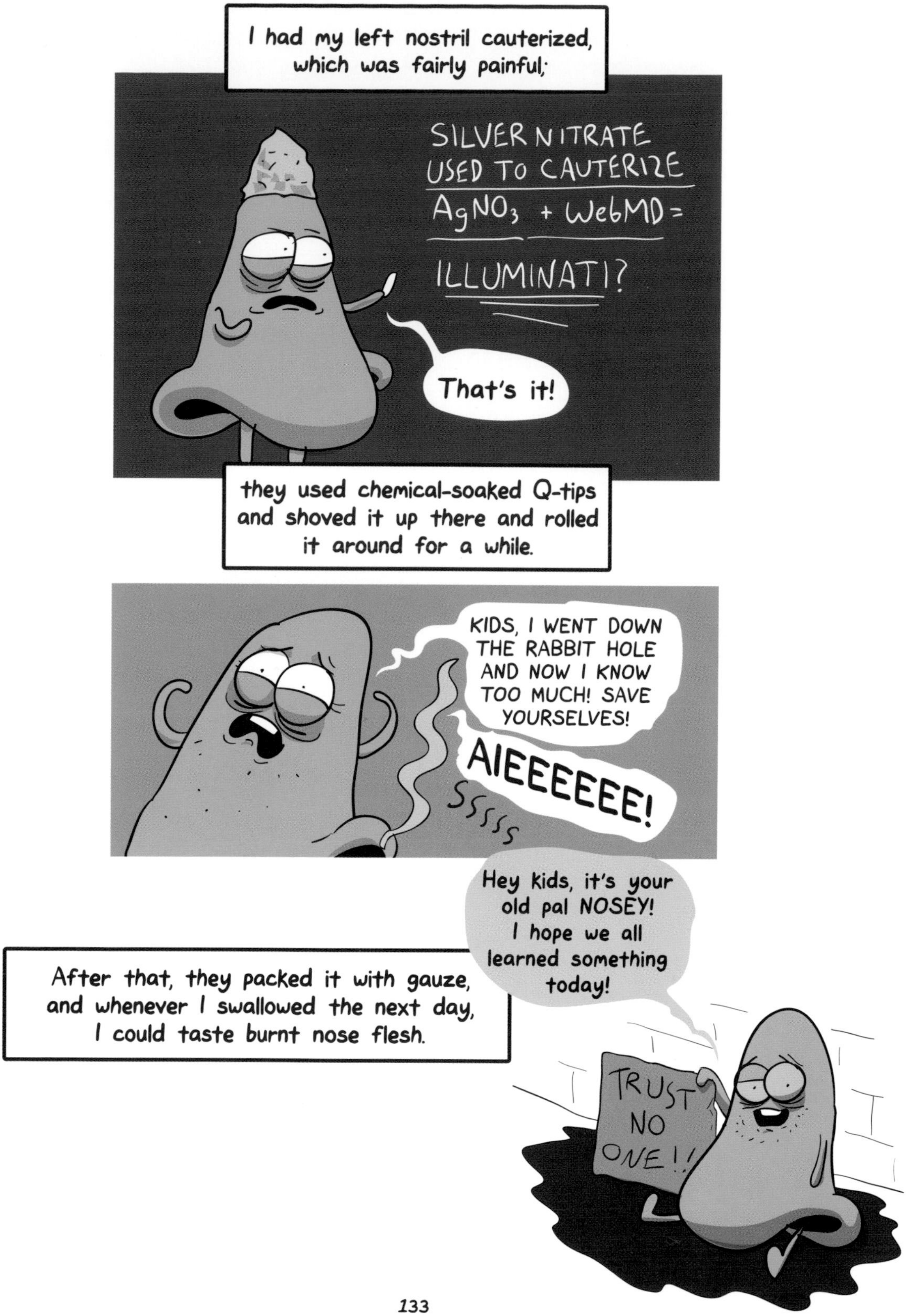

I had my left nostril cauterized, which was fairly painful;
SILVER NITRATE
USED TO CAUTERIZE
$AgNO_3$ + WebMD =
ILLUMINATI?
That's it!
they used chemical-soaked Q-tips and shoved it up there and rolled it around for a while.
KIDS, I WENT DOWN THE RABBIT HOLE AND NOW I KNOW TOO MUCH! SAVE YOURSELVES!
AIEEEEEE!
SSSSS
After that, they packed it with gauze, and whenever I swallowed the next day, I could taste burnt nose flesh.
Hey kids, it's your old pal NOSEY! I hope we all learned something today!
TRUST NO ONE!!

# CHAPTER 20

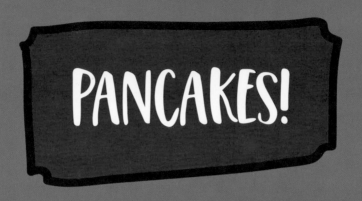

## PANCAKES!

told by Kim Pigford

My dad had taken my mother to the ER with a stomach flu, leaving my younger sister and I to fend for ourselves for dinner.

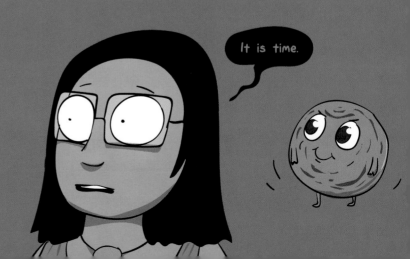

It is time.

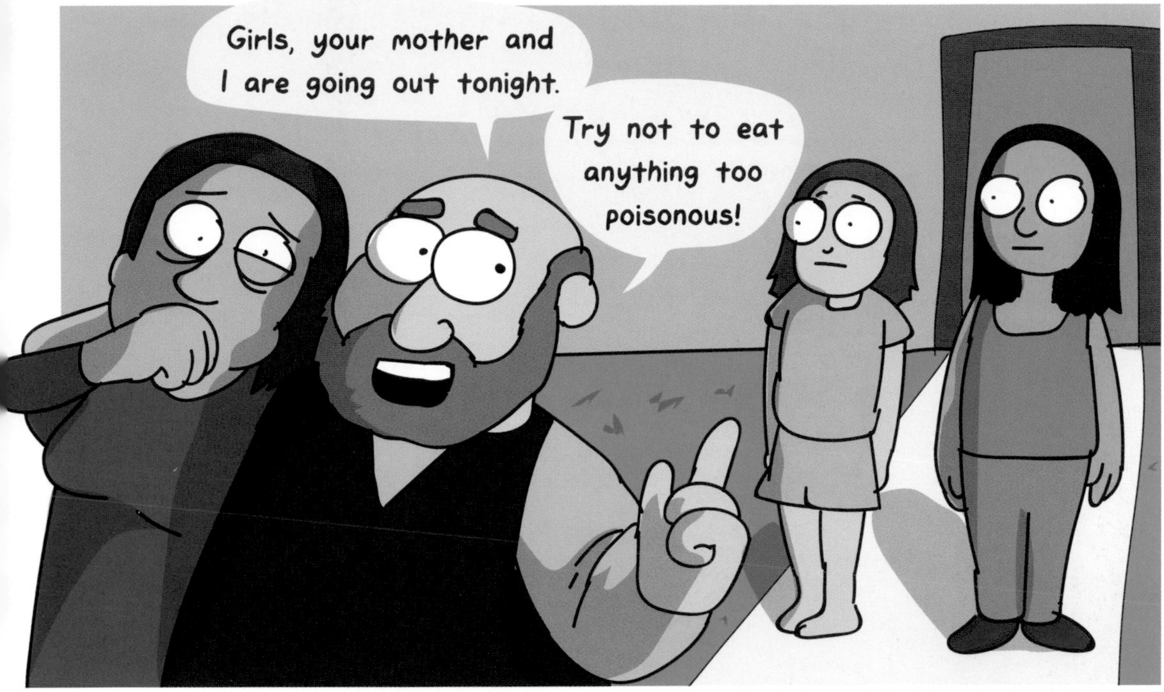
Girls, your mother and I are going out tonight.
Try not to eat anything too poisonous!

We found this old box of pancake mix in the pantry and decided to make pancakes.

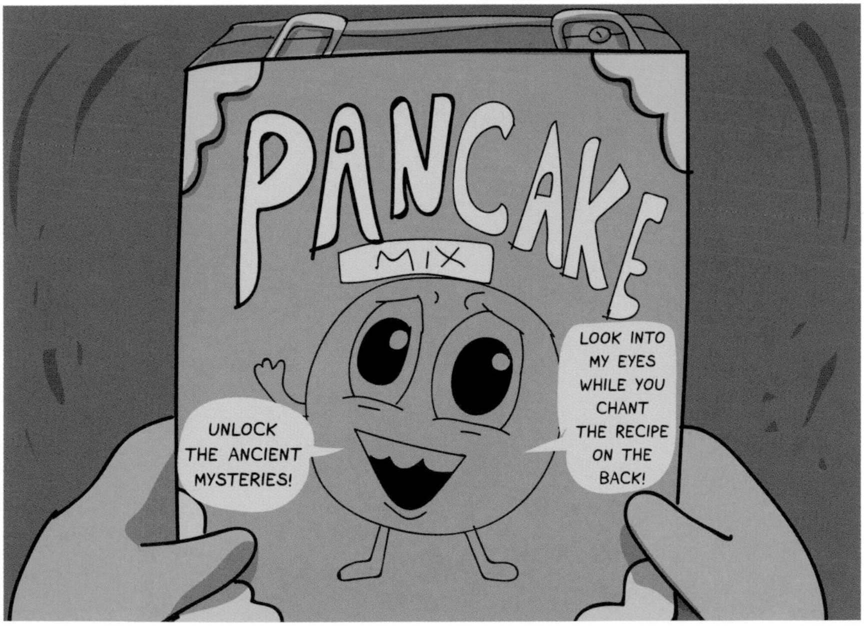
PANCAKE
MIX
UNLOCK THE ANCIENT MYSTERIES!
LOOK INTO MY EYES WHILE YOU CHANT THE RECIPE ON THE BACK!

When my sister opened the box, there was this weird brownish dust on top of the pancake powder that looked like part of the cardboard had disintegrated.

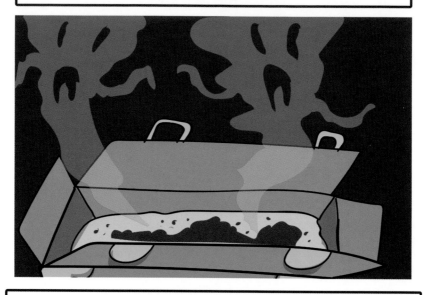

My sister thought we should cook something else, but I figured if we just scooped that part off, we could make pancakes with the mix in the middle of the box.

I'M FREE! THE CURSE IS LIFTED!

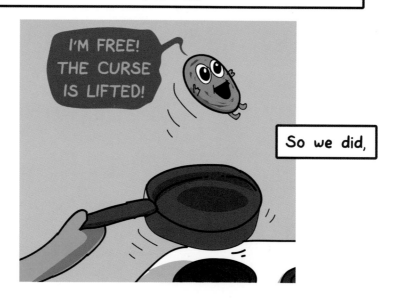

So we did,

and I ate three pancakes,
because I was super hungry.

AH HA HA
YEEESS!

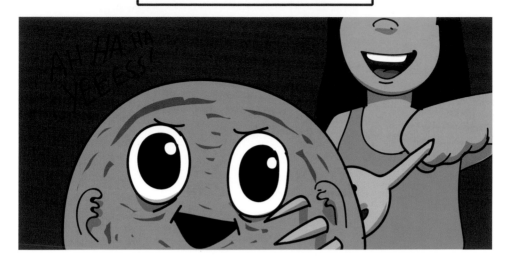

TWENTY MINUTES LATER...

my dad came home with my mom and we were watching TV in the living room. My throat started to get itchy and I started to wheeze a bit.

What a lovely evening!
HHHHH HHHH
STOCKS

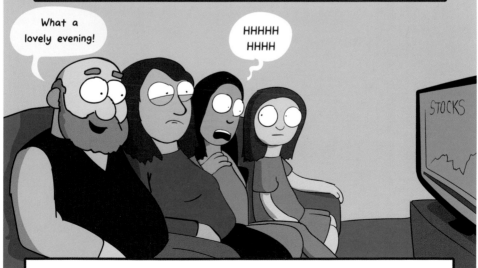

I have allergies, so I went to the bathroom and took a Benadryl and figured I'd be fine in a bit.

# TEN MINUTES LATER...

I was lying disoriented on the couch, struggling to breathe.

My mom was still really drugged from her ER visit and told me to quit breathing the way I was before I made myself sick.

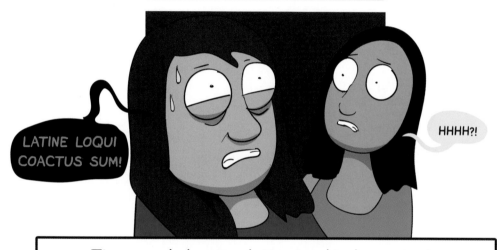

LATINE LOQUI COACTUS SUM!

HHHH?!

Then my dad noticed the trouble I was having and alerted my mom, who asked what we ate for dinner. My sister recounted the pancake story.

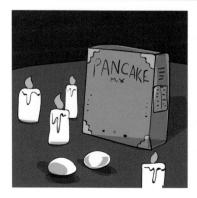

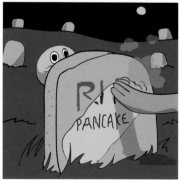

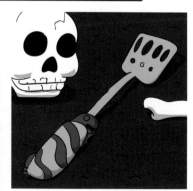

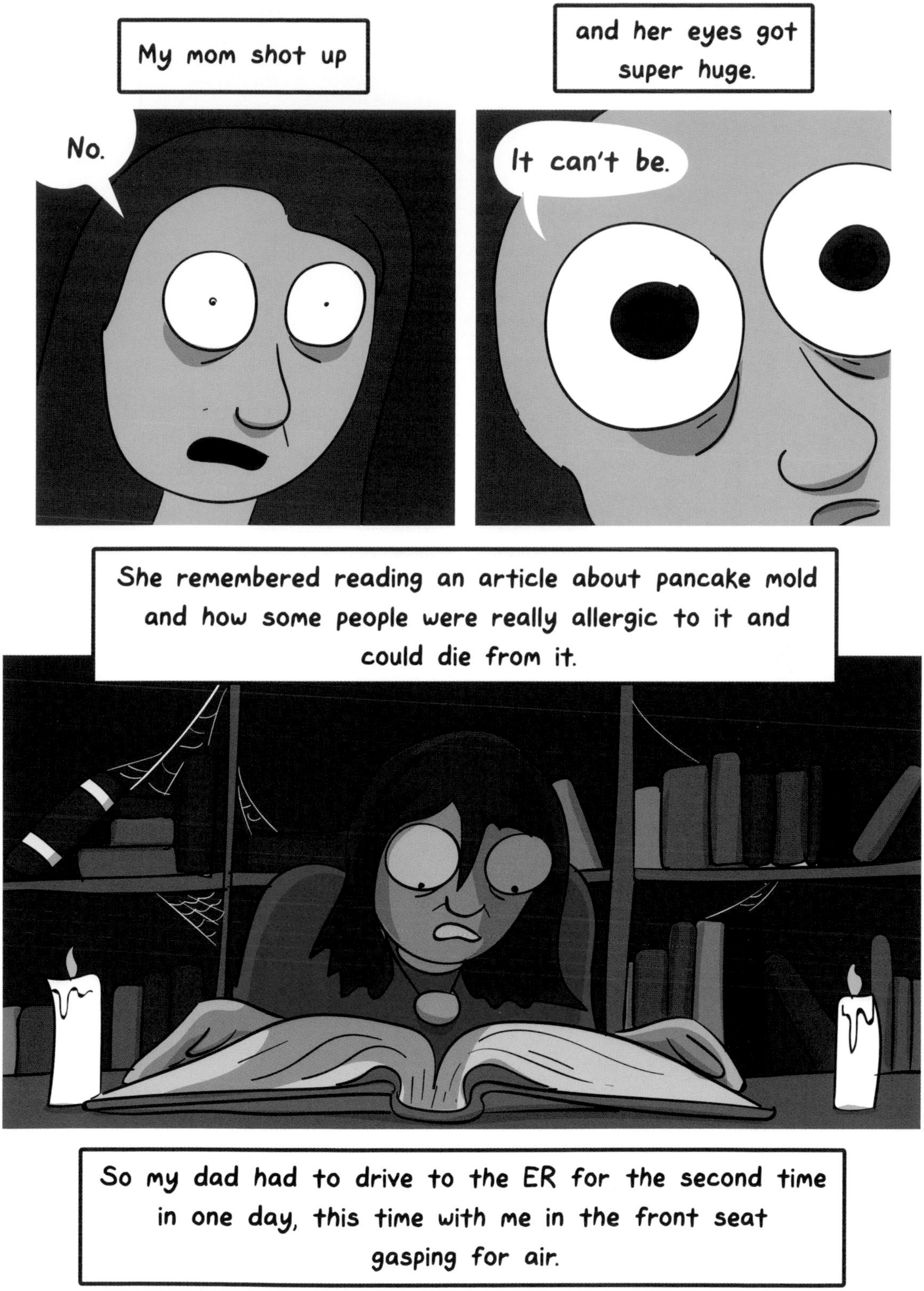

My mom shot up
No.
and her eyes got super huge.
It can't be.
She remembered reading an article about pancake mold and how some people were really allergic to it and could die from it.
So my dad had to drive to the ER for the second time in one day, this time with me in the front seat gasping for air.

When we got to the hospital, the receptionist
asked me if I was having trouble breathing.
I grabbed my throat and continued to wheeze,
which answered her question.

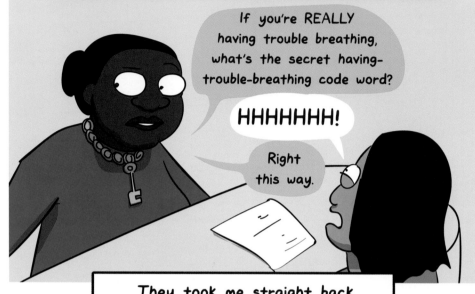

If you're REALLY
having trouble breathing,
what's the secret having-
trouble-breathing code word?

HHHHHHH!

Right
this way.

They took me straight back,
leaving my dad to do the paperwork.

I think this must have been this particular nurse's
first night on the job or something because
he was really young.

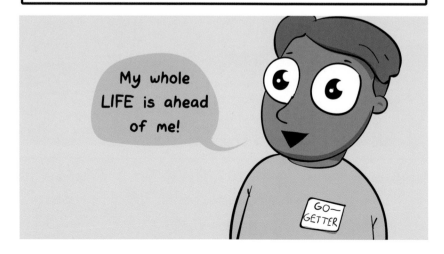

My whole
LIFE is ahead
of me!

GO-
GETTER

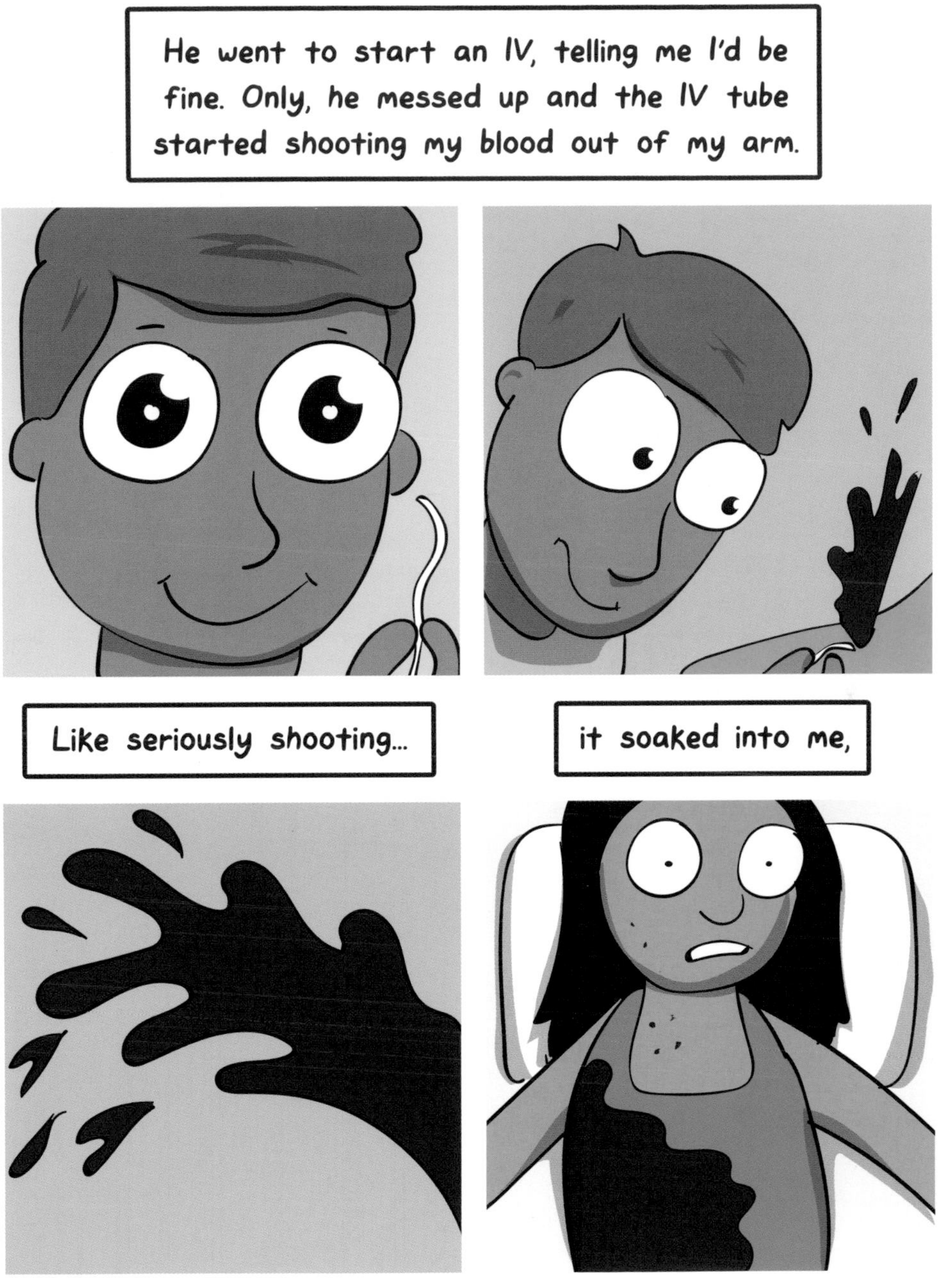
He went to start an IV, telling me I'd be fine. Only, he messed up and the IV tube started shooting my blood out of my arm.
Like seriously shooting...
it soaked into me,

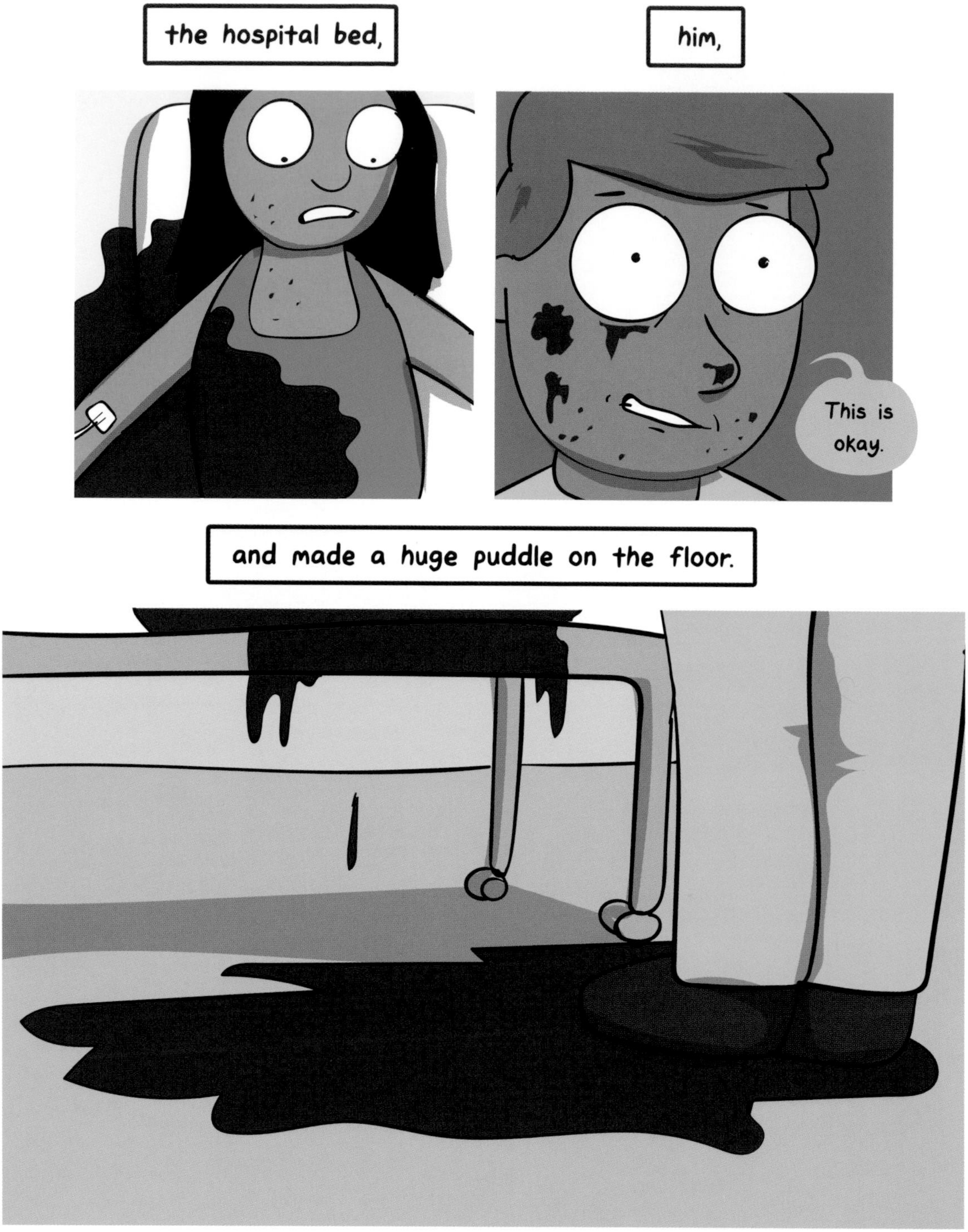
the hospital bed,
him,
This is okay.
and made a huge puddle on the floor.

He apologized and tried to fix it.

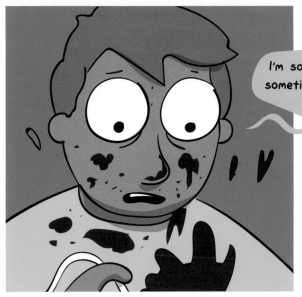

I'm so sorry; I swear, sometimes this doesn't happen!

Meanwhile,

my stomach, realizing the perpetrator of my current distress was residing inside it, decided to rebel and prepared to eject its contents back the way they came.

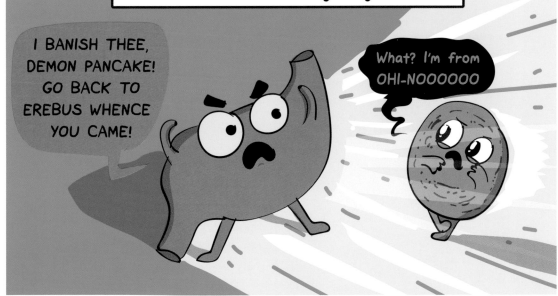

I BANISH THEE, DEMON PANCAKE! GO BACK TO EREBUS WHENCE YOU CAME!

What? I'm from OHI-NOOOOOO

I got really panicky and told the nurse I felt like I was going to throw up.

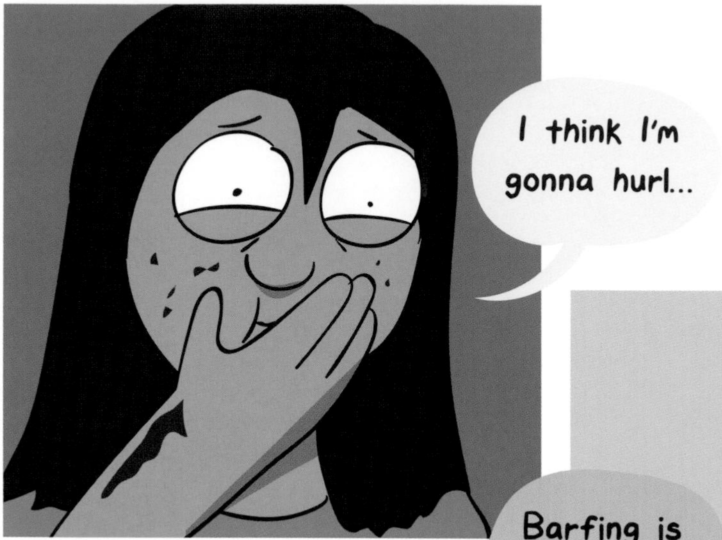
I think I'm gonna hurl...

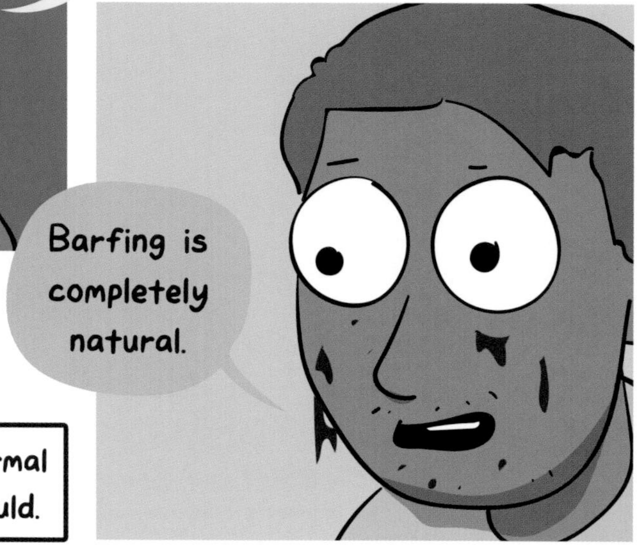
Barfing is completely natural.

He said that's normal and I probably would.

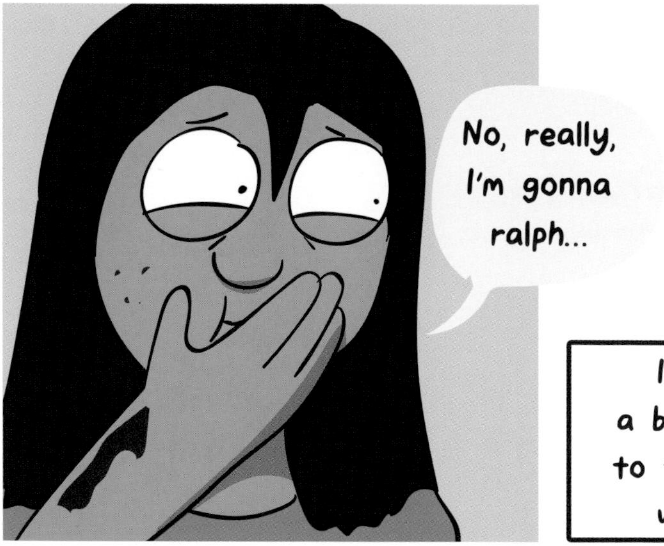
No, really, I'm gonna ralph...

I told him, no, I need a bucket now or I'm going to throw up on your head while you fix this IV.

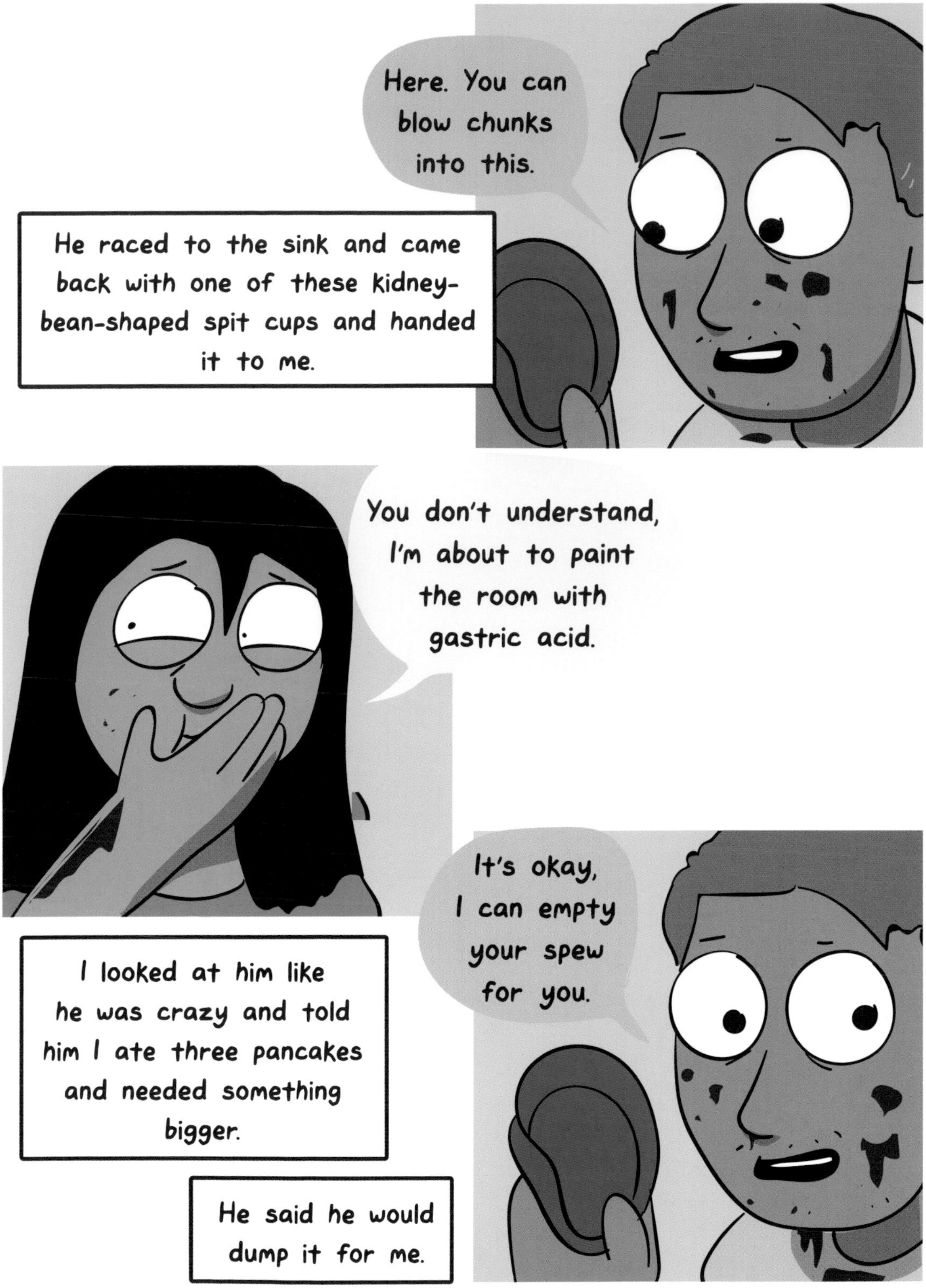
Here. You can blow chunks into this.
He raced to the sink and came back with one of these kidney-bean-shaped spit cups and handed it to me.
You don't understand, I'm about to paint the room with gastric acid.
I looked at him like he was crazy and told him I ate three pancakes and needed something bigger.
It's okay, I can empty your spew for you.
He said he would dump it for me.

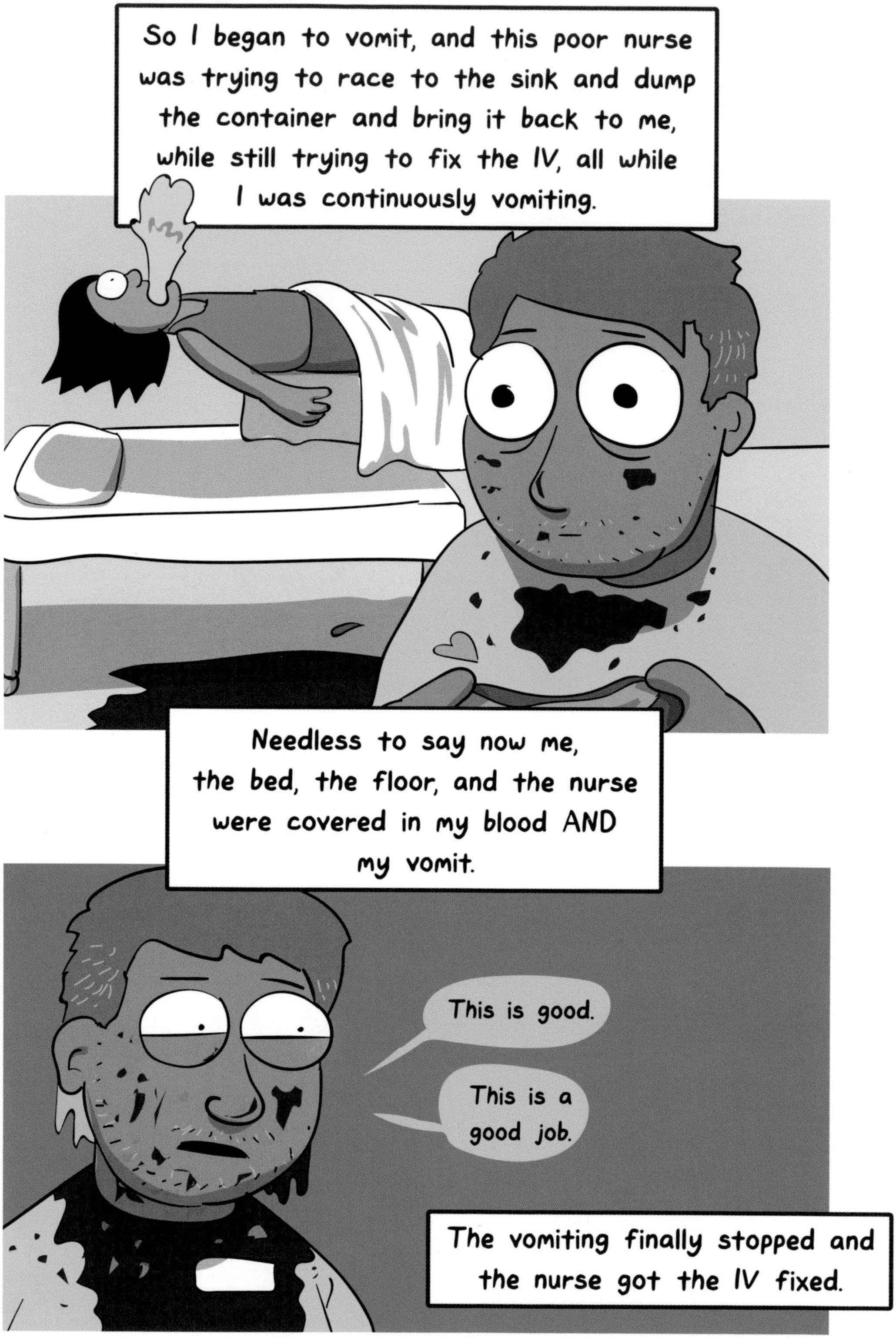
So I began to vomit, and this poor nurse was trying to race to the sink and dump the container and bring it back to me, while still trying to fix the IV, all while I was continuously vomiting.
Needless to say now me, the bed, the floor, and the nurse were covered in my blood AND my vomit.
This is good.
This is a good job.
The vomiting finally stopped and the nurse got the IV fixed.

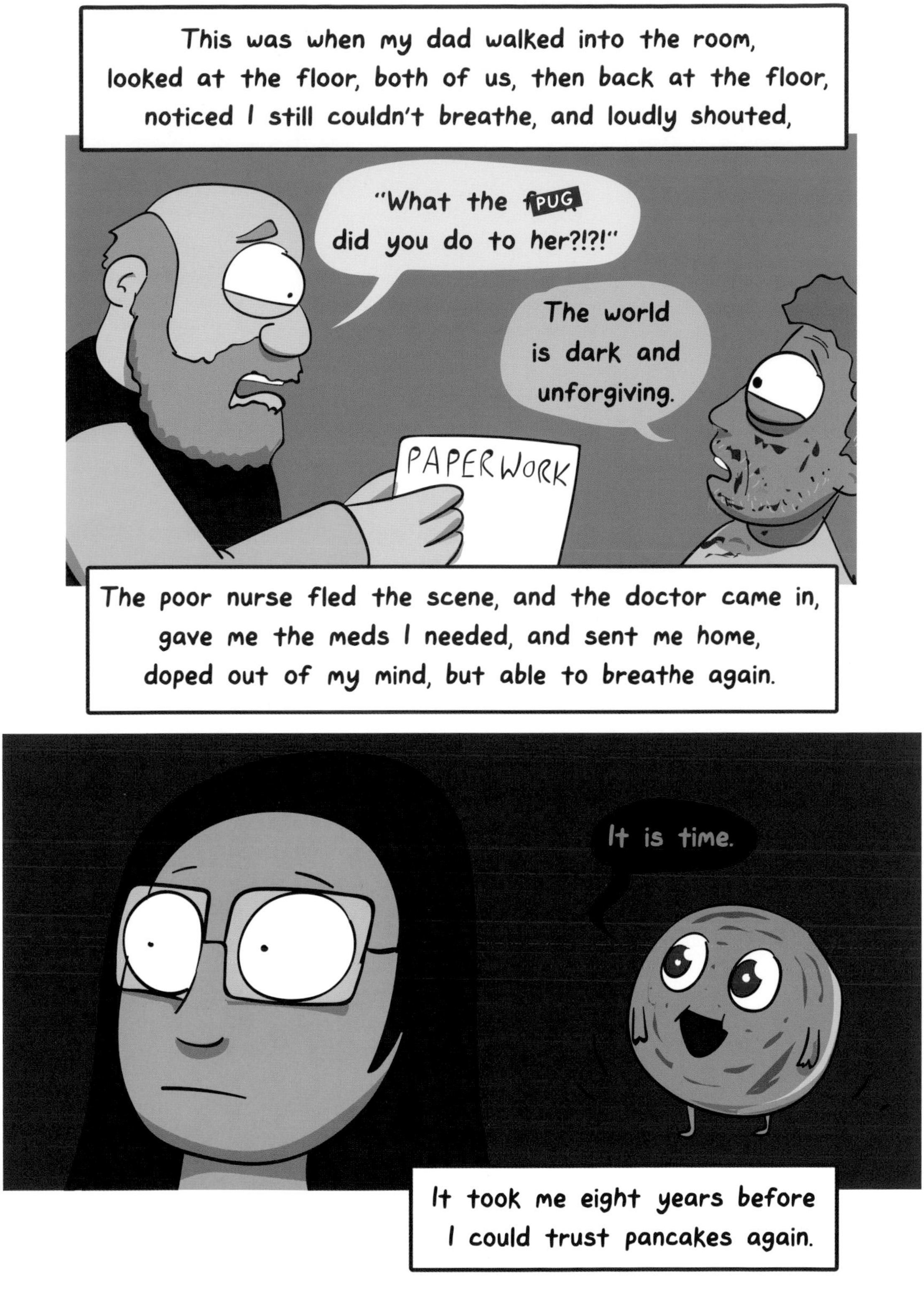
This was when my dad walked into the room, looked at the floor, both of us, then back at the floor, noticed I still couldn't breathe, and loudly shouted,
"What the fPUG did you do to her?!?!"
The world is dark and unforgiving.
PAPERWORK
The poor nurse fled the scene, and the doctor came in, gave me the meds I needed, and sent me home, doped out of my mind, but able to breathe again.
It is time.
It took me eight years before I could trust pancakes again.

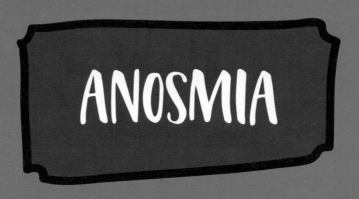

# CHAPTER 21

# ANOSMIA

told by Frank C.

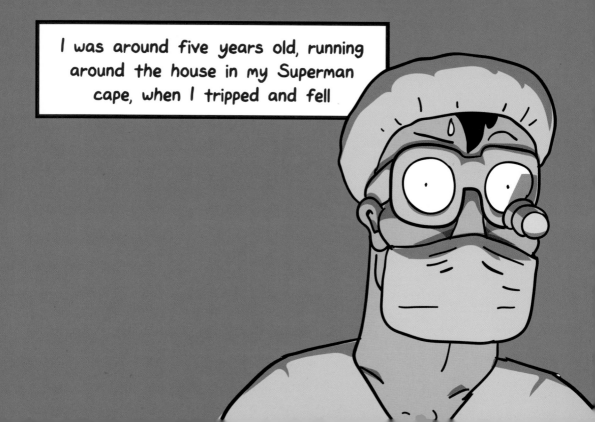

I was around five years old, running around the house in my Superman cape, when I tripped and fell

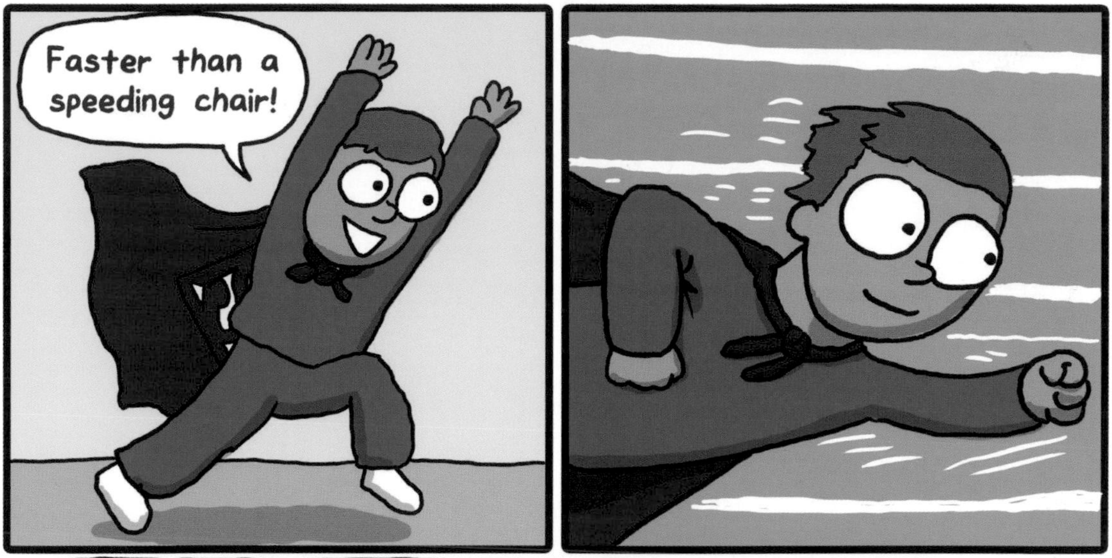
Faster than a speeding chair!

and hit my head on the edge of a chair.
Off to the ER I went, and stitches were the final result.

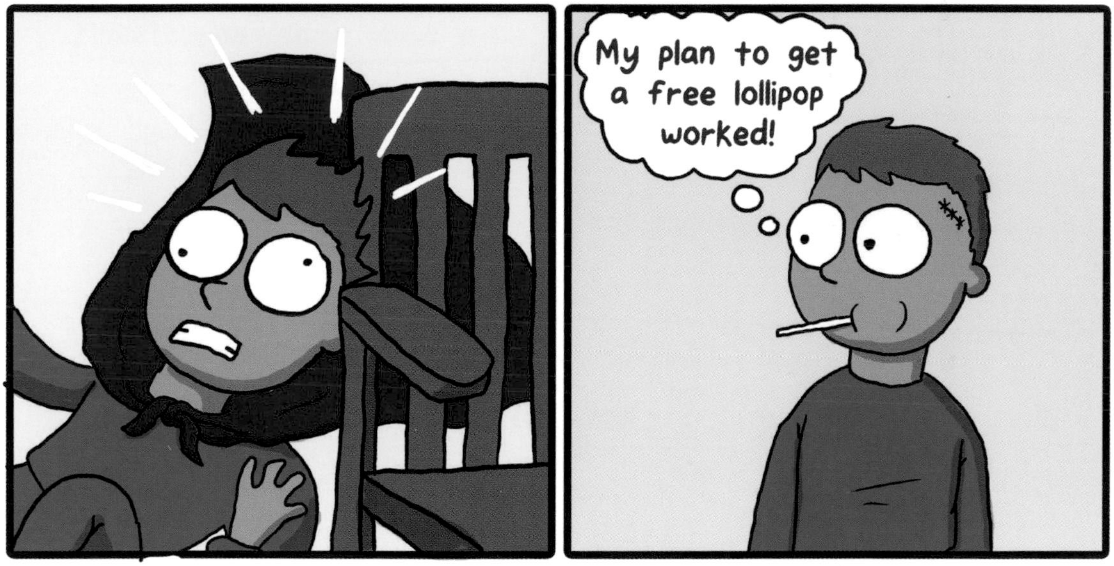
My plan to get a free lollipop worked!

Well, that was pretty boring, right?

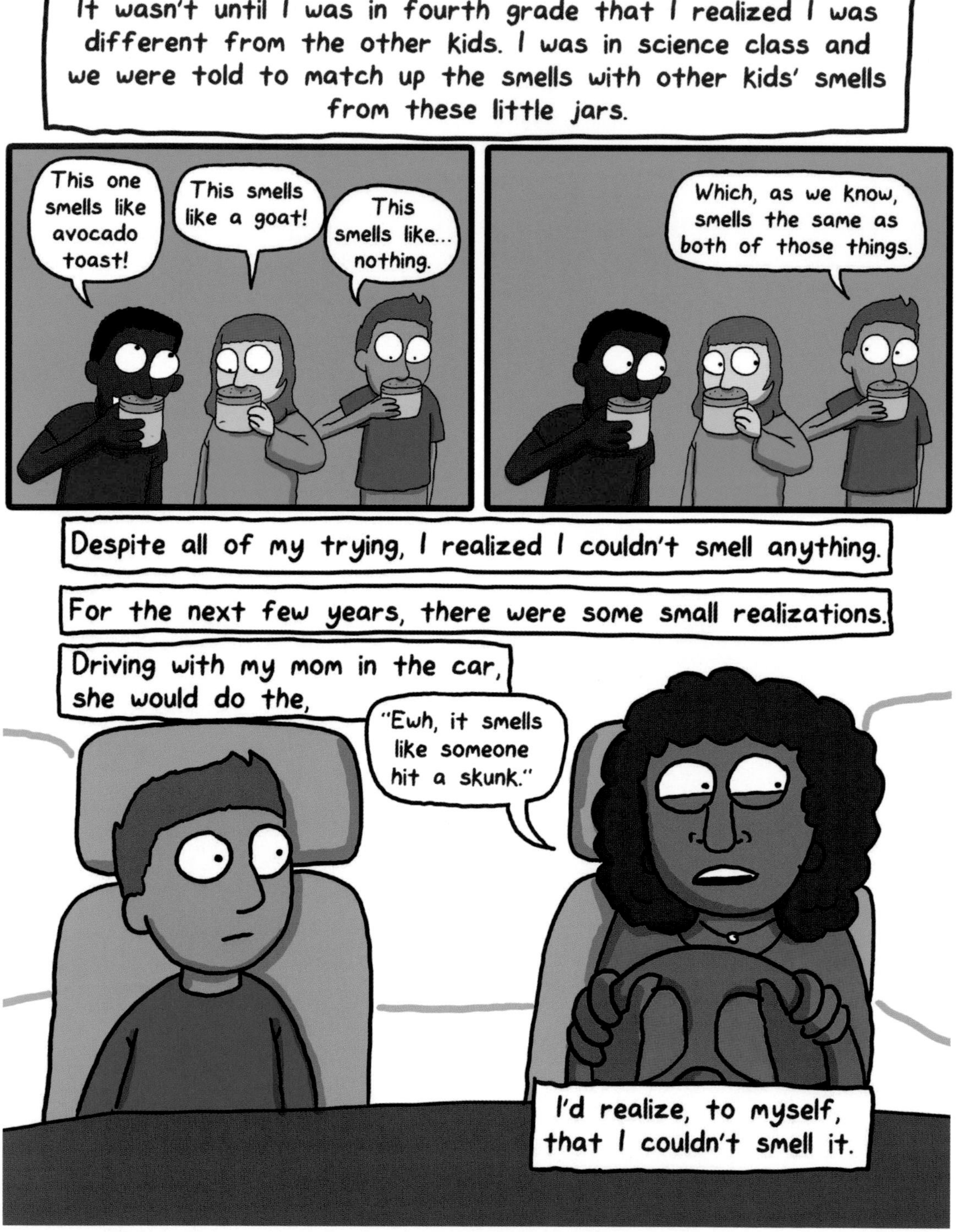
It wasn't until I was in fourth grade that I realized I was different from the other kids. I was in science class and we were told to match up the smells with other kids' smells from these little jars.
This one smells like avocado toast!
This smells like a goat!
This smells like... nothing.
Which, as we know, smells the same as both of those things.
Despite all of my trying, I realized I couldn't smell anything.
For the next few years, there were some small realizations.
Driving with my mom in the car, she would do the,
"Ewh, it smells like someone hit a skunk."
I'd realize, to myself, that I couldn't smell it.

People have a tendency to be like,

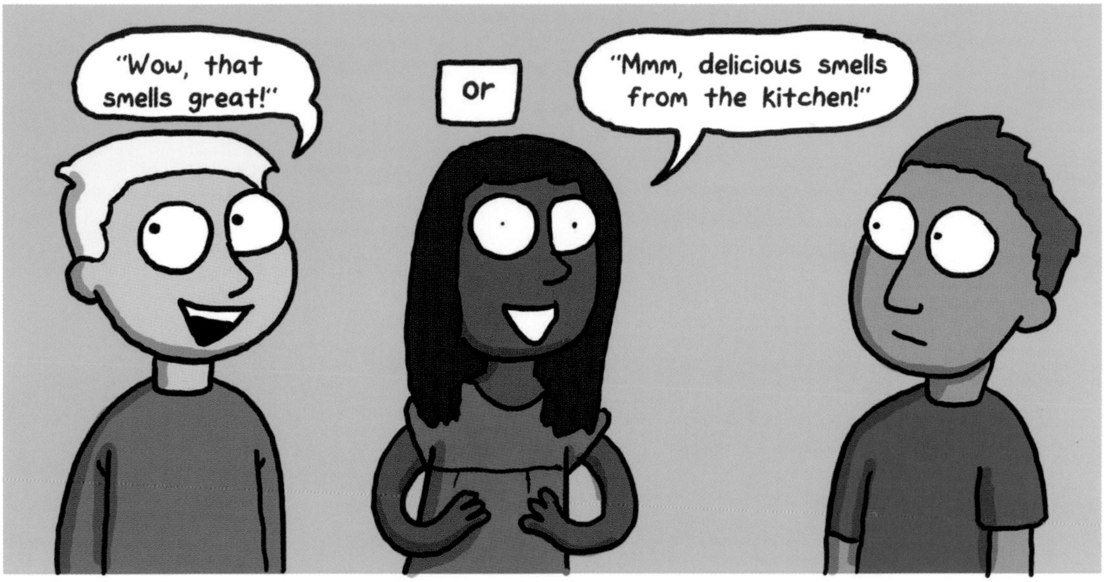
"Wow, that smells great!"
or
"Mmm, delicious smells from the kitchen!"

When you're a kid, you mostly just agree until you realize you have no idea what they're talking about.

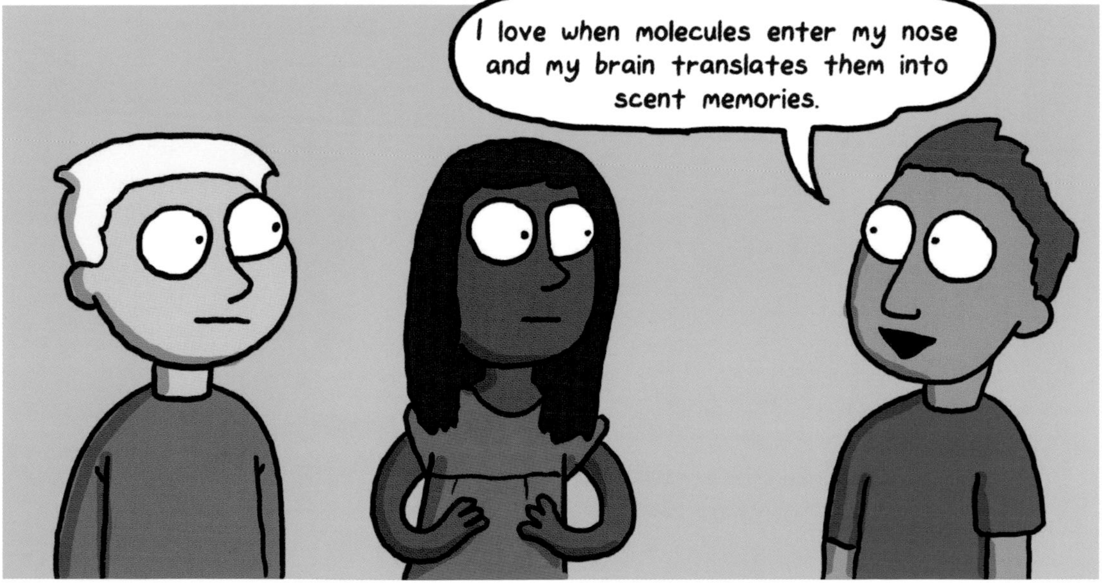
I love when molecules enter my nose and my brain translates them into scent memories.

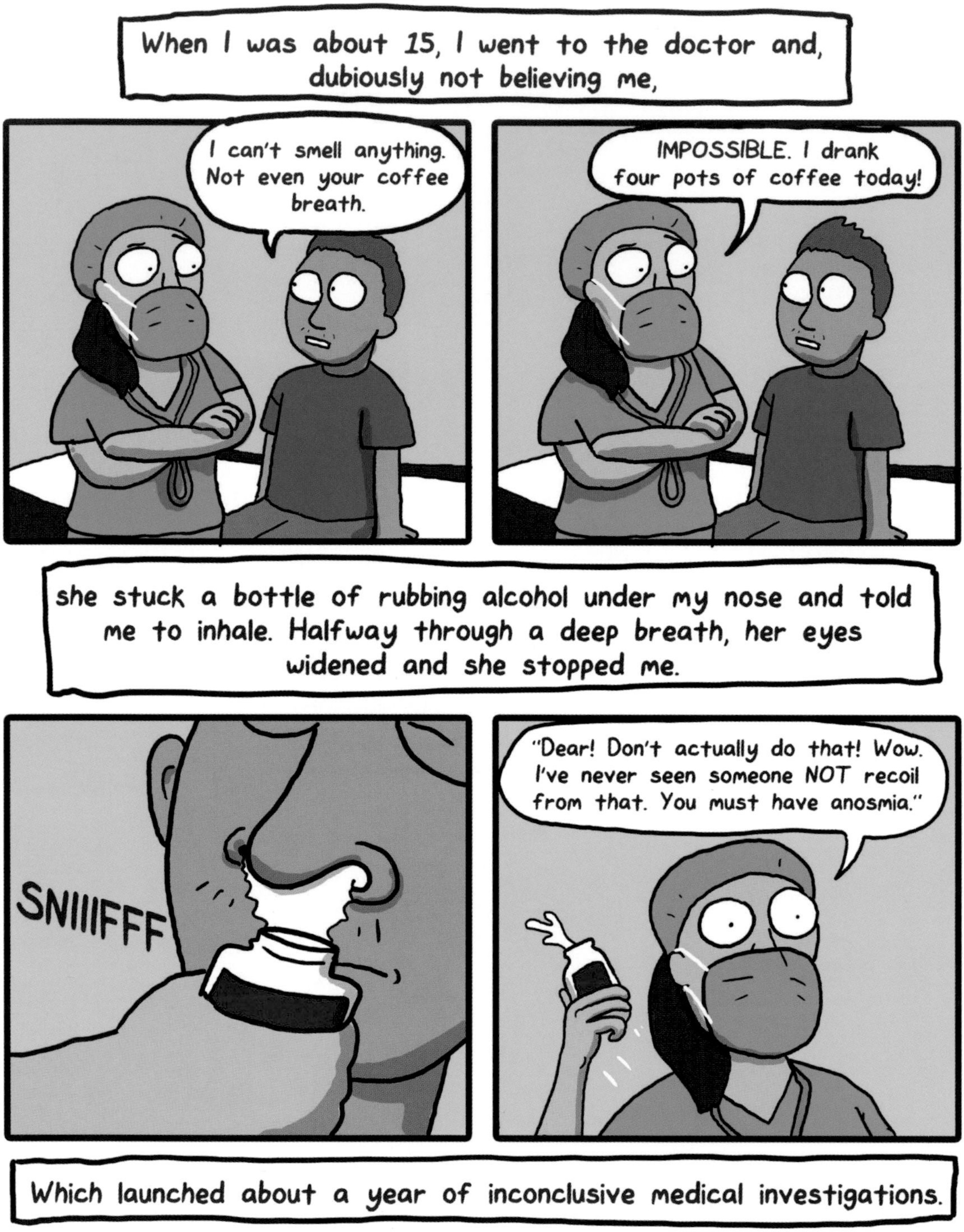

When I was about 15, I went to the doctor and, dubiously not believing me,
I can't smell anything. Not even your coffee breath.
IMPOSSIBLE. I drank four pots of coffee today!
she stuck a bottle of rubbing alcohol under my nose and told me to inhale. Halfway through a deep breath, her eyes widened and she stopped me.
SNIIIFFF
"Dear! Don't actually do that! Wow. I've never seen someone NOT recoil from that. You must have anosmia."
Which launched about a year of inconclusive medical investigations.

And hence, as an adult, I still can't smell.

I still just nod and smile when someone says how great that food smells at a restaurant.

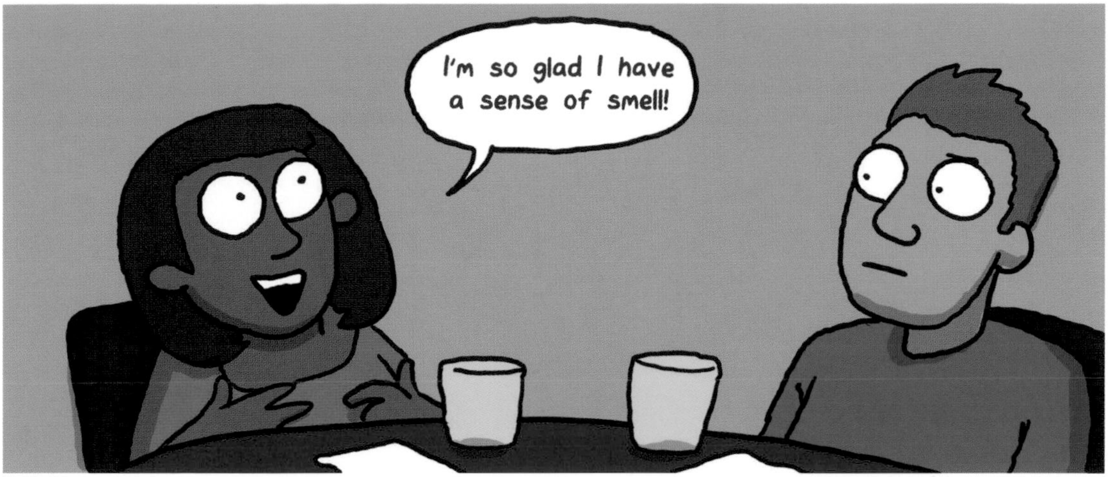
I'm so glad I have a sense of smell!

Or how bad the rats and garbage smell in New York City...

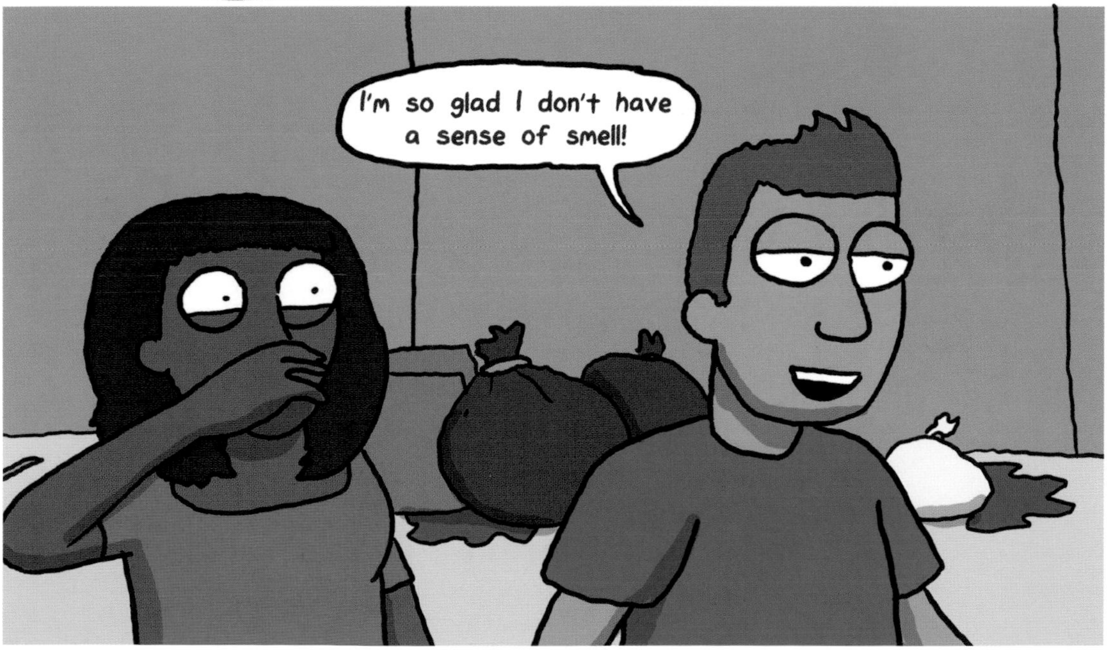
I'm so glad I don't have a sense of smell!

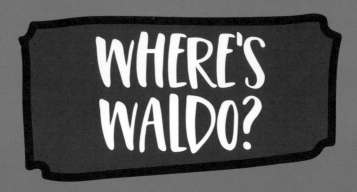

# CHAPTER 22

# WHERE'S WALDO?

told by Jessica Gumkowski

I'm a 22-year-old female with a weird and rather rare condition called situs ambiguus polysplenia—

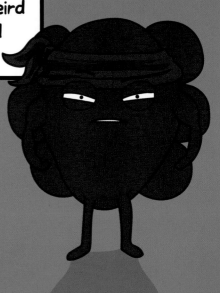

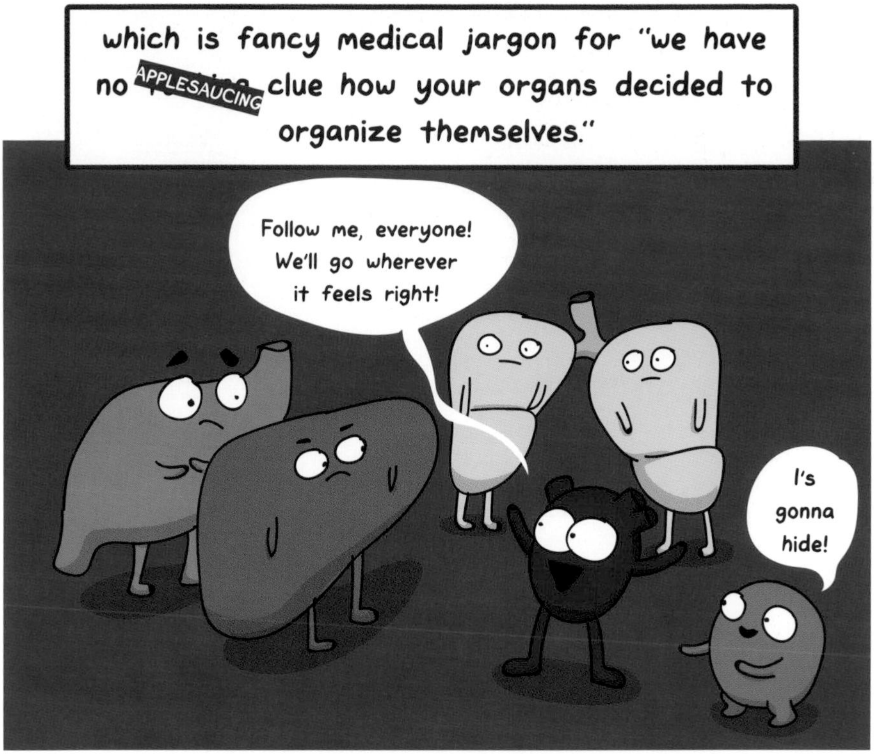
which is fancy medical jargon for "we have no APPLESAUCING clue how your organs decided to organize themselves."
Follow me, everyone! We'll go wherever it feels right!
I's gonna hide!

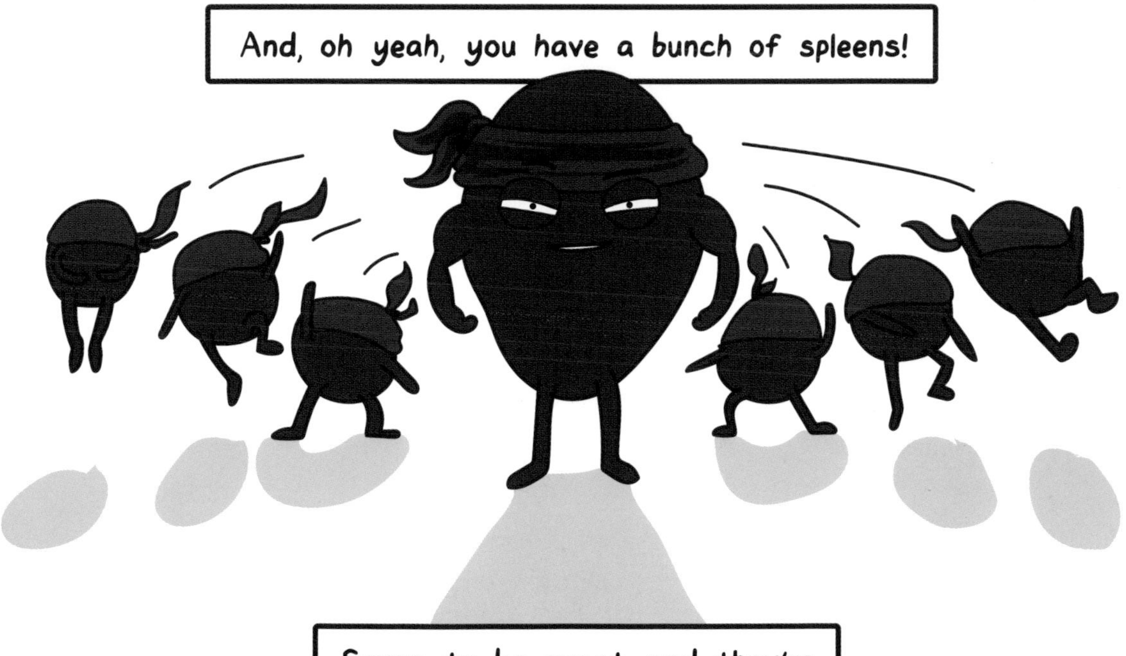
And, oh yeah, you have a bunch of spleens!
Seven to be exact, and they're referred to as splenules.

Anyway, you'd assume this would be the kind of thing doctors would notice when a baby is born.

Nope!

Eight cartoon fingers, eight cartoon toes, two eyes, a slab of hair, probably one spleen, presumably organs in the right spots.

SHE'S PERFECT!

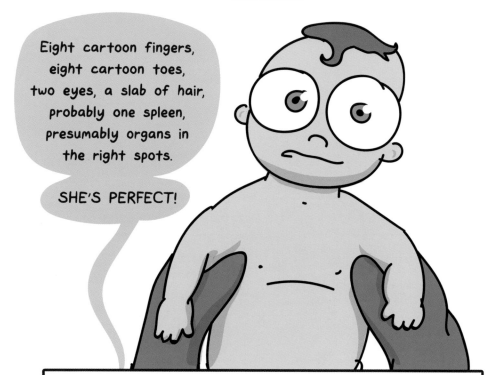

Apparently, I was too adorable, and corners were cut or something. I grew up sick, but my parents always had a "rub some dirt on it!" attitude, so we never investigated further.

I stubbed my toe!
Rub some dirt on it.
My tummy hurts!
Rub some dirt on it.
I need help with my homework!
Rub some dirt on it.
I got dirt in my eyes!
Rub some dirt on it.


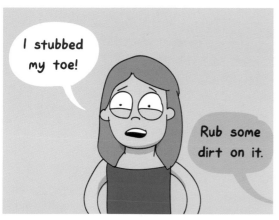

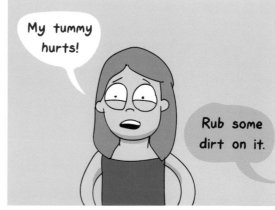

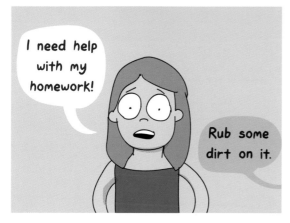

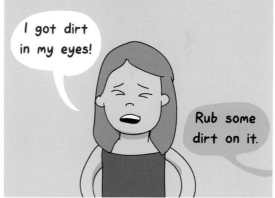

Somehow, and doctors seriously don't know how, I lived with the different complications of situs ambiguus. In fact, it wasn't until I was 18 that we even knew I had it at all.

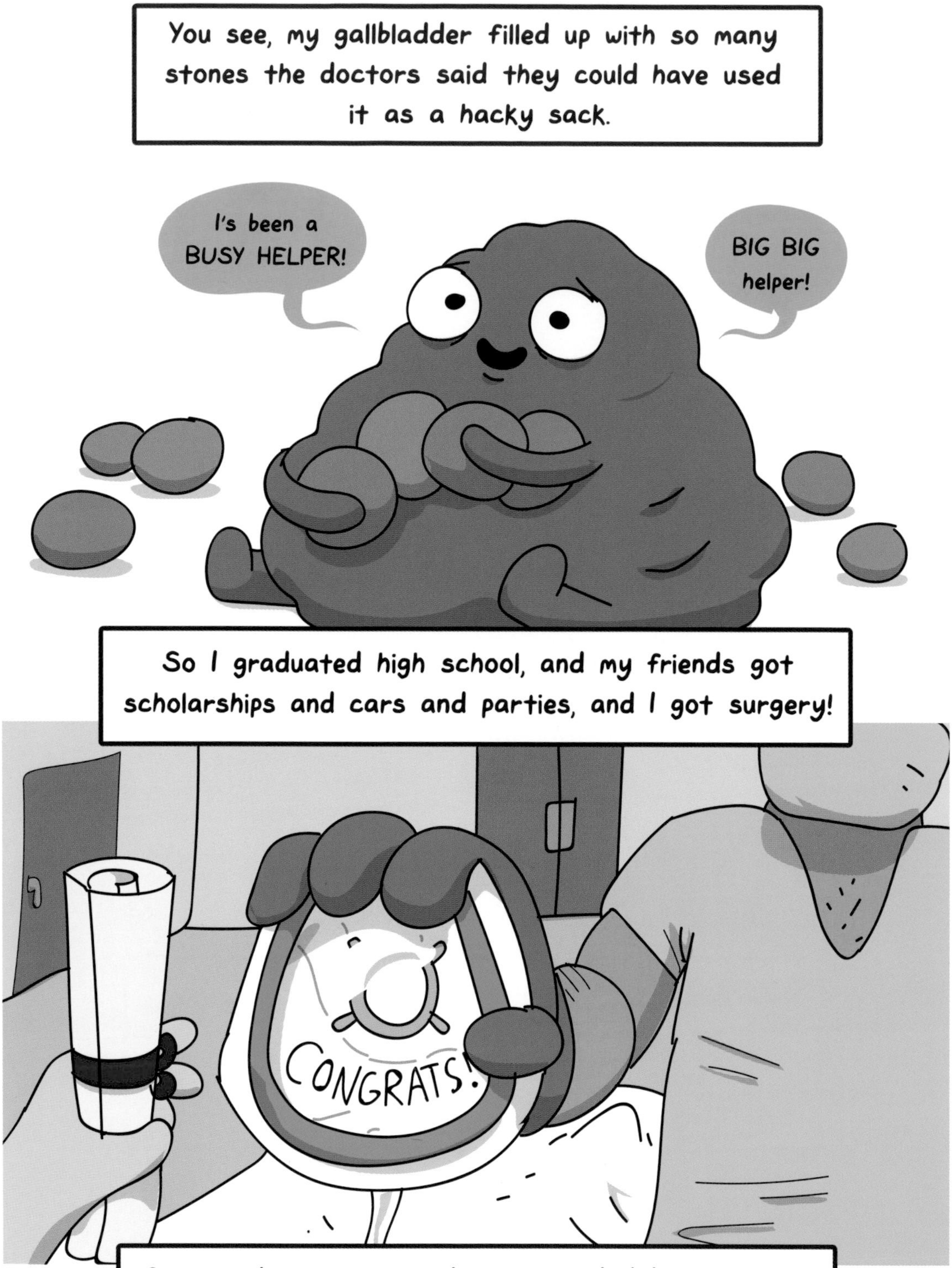
You see, my gallbladder filled up with so many stones the doctors said they could have used it as a hacky sack.
I's been a BUSY HELPER!
BIG BIG helper!
So I graduated high school, and my friends got scholarships and cars and parties, and I got surgery!
CONGRATS!
So the doctors prepped me up and did their thing.

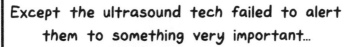

Except the ultrasound tech failed to alert them to something very important...

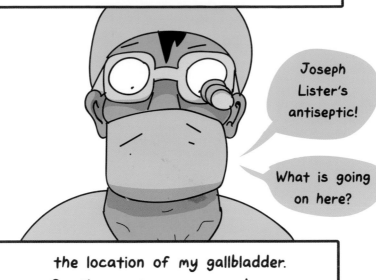

Joseph Lister's antiseptic!

What is going on here?

the location of my gallbladder. So they cut me open and were baffled as APPLESAUCE

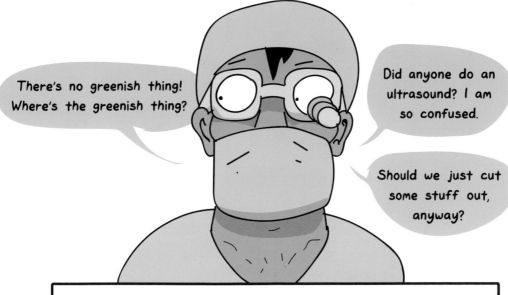

There's no greenish thing! Where's the greenish thing?

Did anyone do an ultrasound? I am so confused.

Should we just cut some stuff out, anyway?

You see, in my particular case of situs ambiguus, my gallbladder is actually on my right (anatomical left).

## LEFT ISOMERISM (polysplenia)

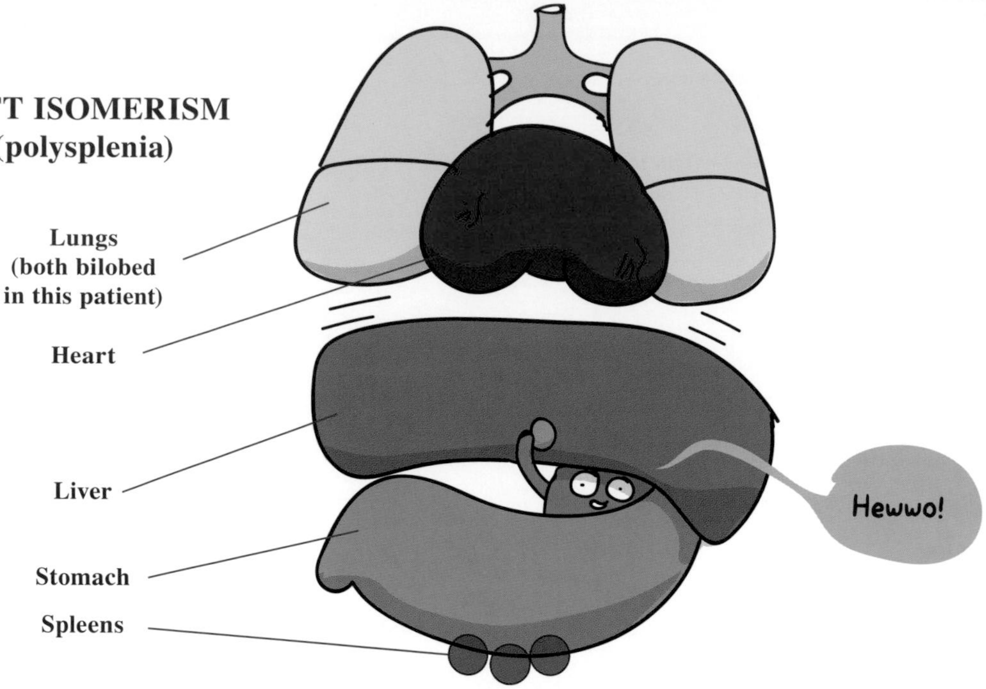
Lungs
(both bilobed
in this patient)
Heart
Liver
Stomach
Spleens
Hewwo!

So needless to say, the surgery became a little more complicated as doctors started playing a game of Where's Waldo during my surgery.

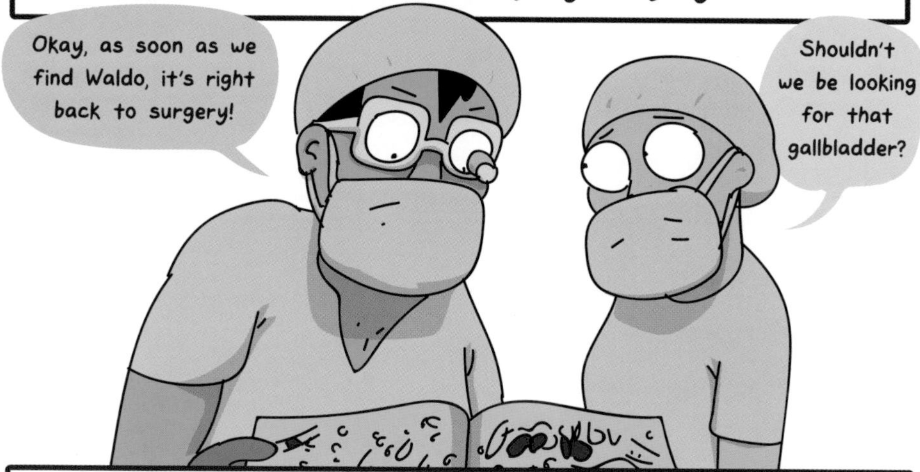
Okay, as soon as we find Waldo, it's right back to surgery!
Shouldn't we be looking for that gallbladder?

A while later, they came out and spoke to my parents. At this point, they were geeking out hard. They told my parents I was, I POO you not, weird. I was medically diagnosed as weird. Thanks, doc.

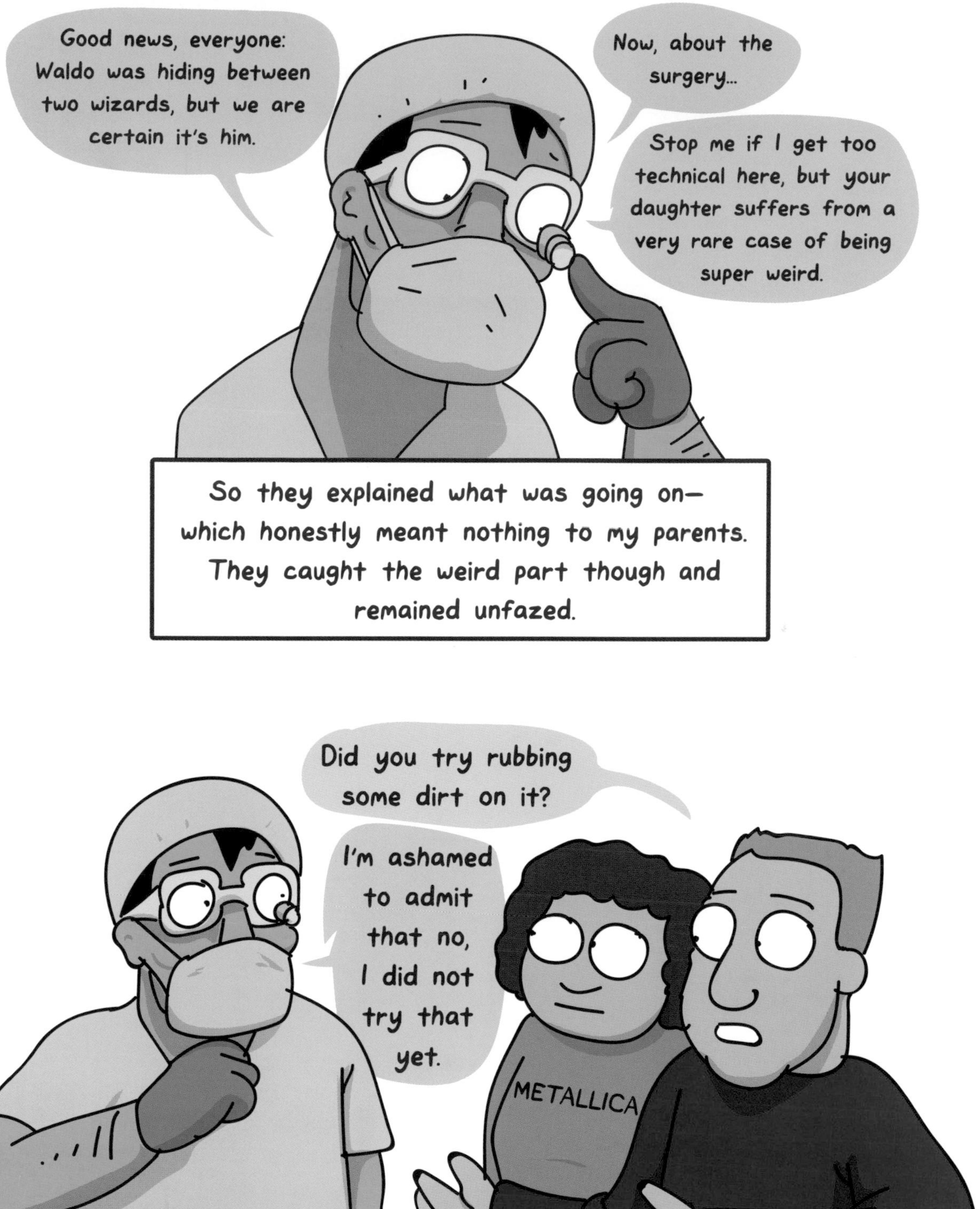
Good news, everyone: Waldo was hiding between two wizards, but we are certain it's him.
Now, about the surgery...
Stop me if I get too technical here, but your daughter suffers from a very rare case of being super weird.
So they explained what was going on—which honestly meant nothing to my parents. They caught the weird part though and remained unfazed.
Did you try rubbing some dirt on it?
I'm ashamed to admit that no, I did not try that yet.
METALLICA

So, long story short, a quick-and-easy walkout procedure turned into a weeklong stay in the hospital, recovering from some very confused and excited doctors poking around my abdomen. I was pretty famous with the staff for that week though, and being a medical student myself now, let me just say, mentioning my condition is better than a pickup line.

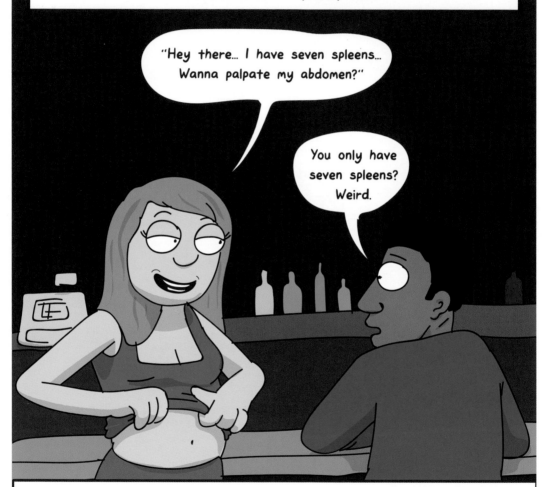

"Hey there... I have seven spleens... Wanna palpate my abdomen?"

You only have seven spleens? Weird.

But it is annoying, too, because many doctors don't know what it is, or the complications. I went to a gastroenterologist who argued with me that I was wrong and I had situs inversus, which is much more manageable.

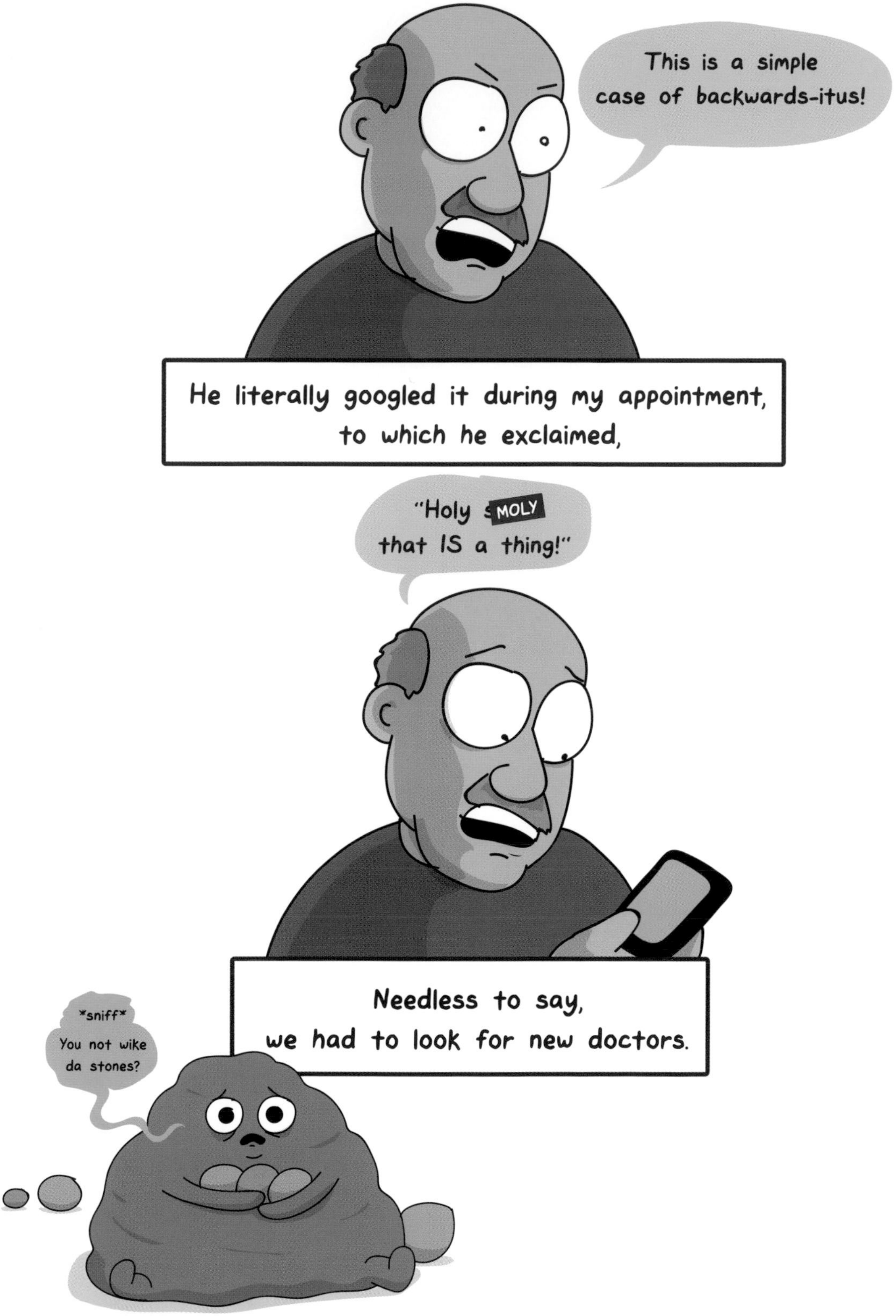
This is a simple case of backwards-itus!
He literally googled it during my appointment, to which he exclaimed,
"Holy sMOLY that IS a thing!"
Needless to say, we had to look for new doctors.
*sniff* You not wike da stones?

# CHAPTER 23

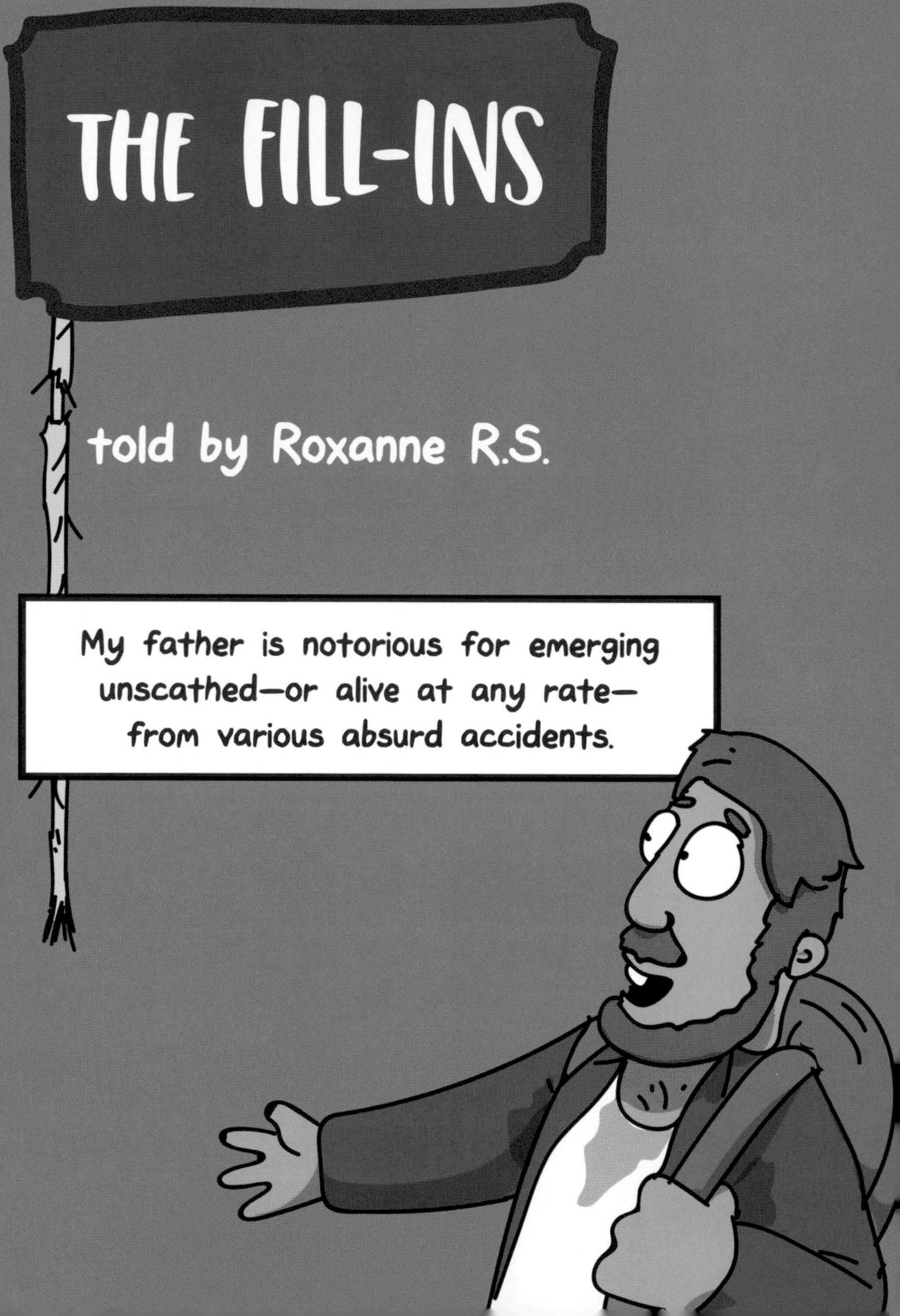
THE FILL-INS
told by Roxanne R.S.
My father is notorious for emerging unscathed—or alive at any rate—from various absurd accidents.

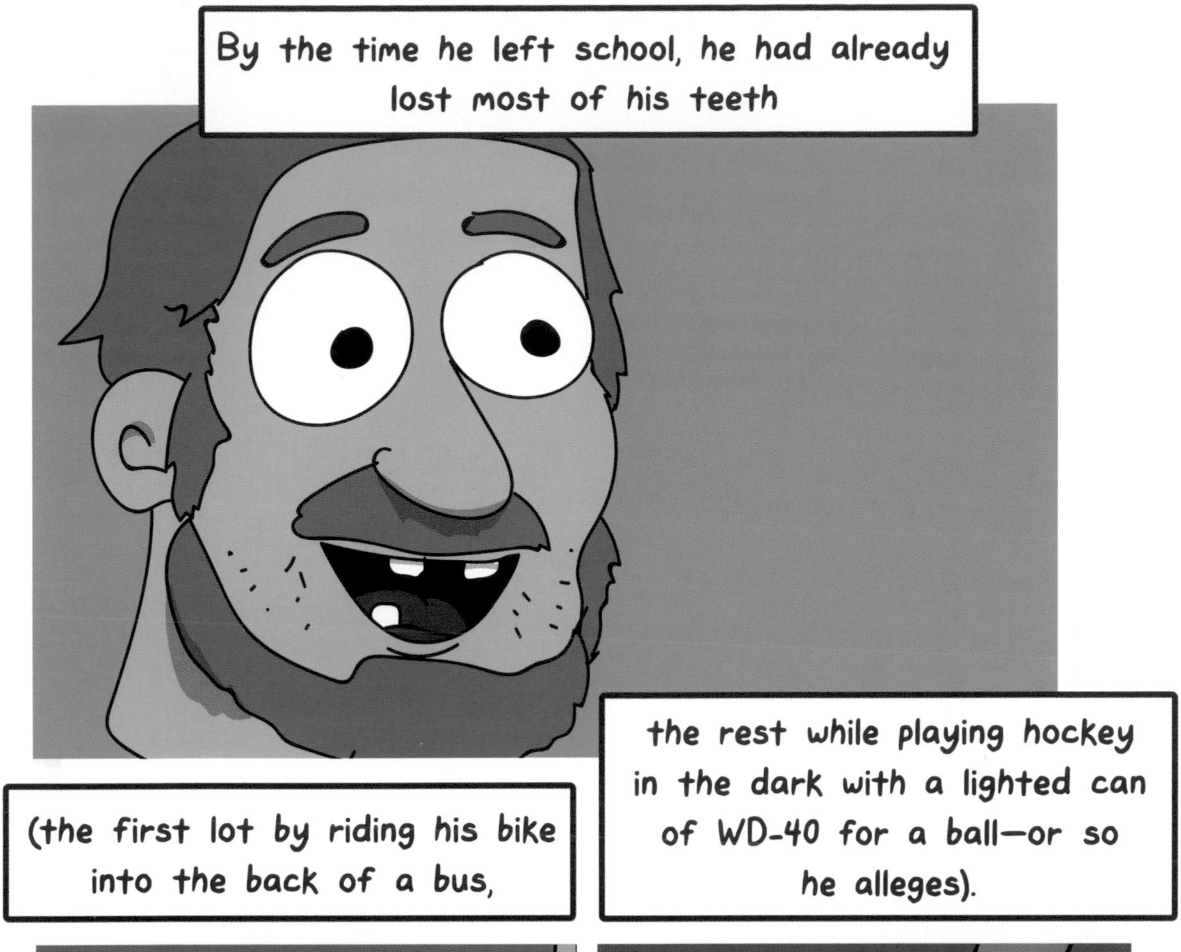
By the time he left school, he had already lost most of his teeth
(the first lot by riding his bike into the back of a bus,
the rest while playing hockey in the dark with a lighted can of WD-40 for a ball—or so he alleges).
SLAM! SLAM!
Bet I can block your shot with my face!
WD-40
You're on!

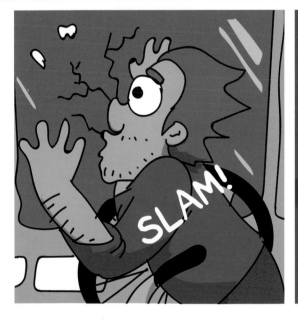

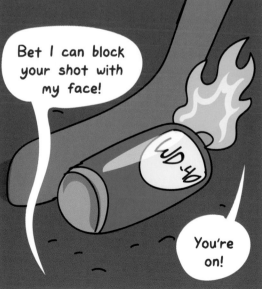

This particular incident took place on the island of St. Helena, where anything can happen. (Absolutely anything.)

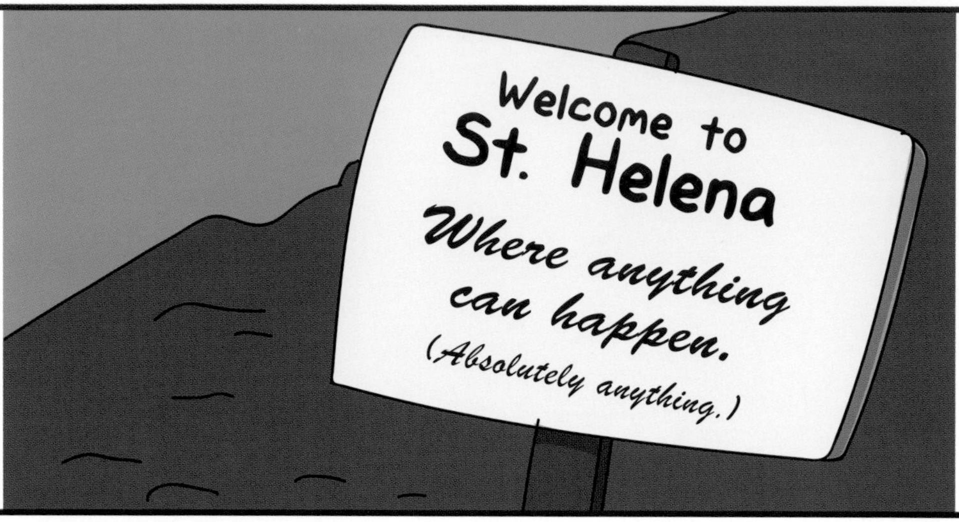
Welcome to
St. Helena
Where anything can happen.
(Absolutely anything.)

So, we were returning from a hike to the other side of the island. The return trip involved climbing up a fairly high cliff, over the edge of which someone had long before fastened a thin piece of rope, now tattered and weather-worn.

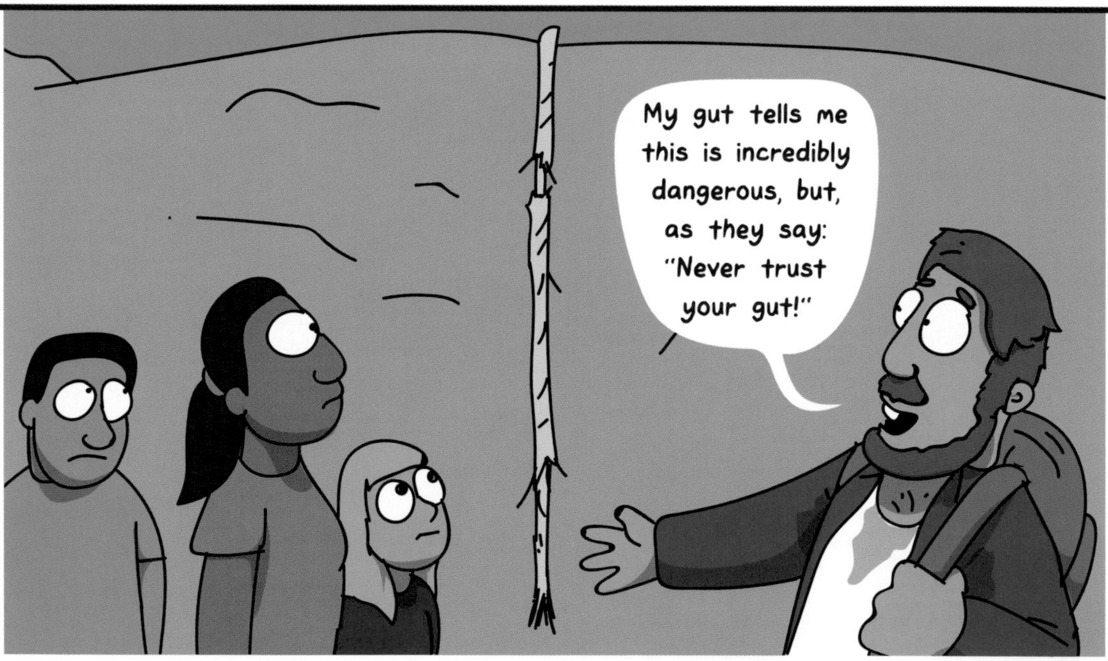
My gut tells me this is incredibly dangerous, but, as they say: "Never trust your gut!"

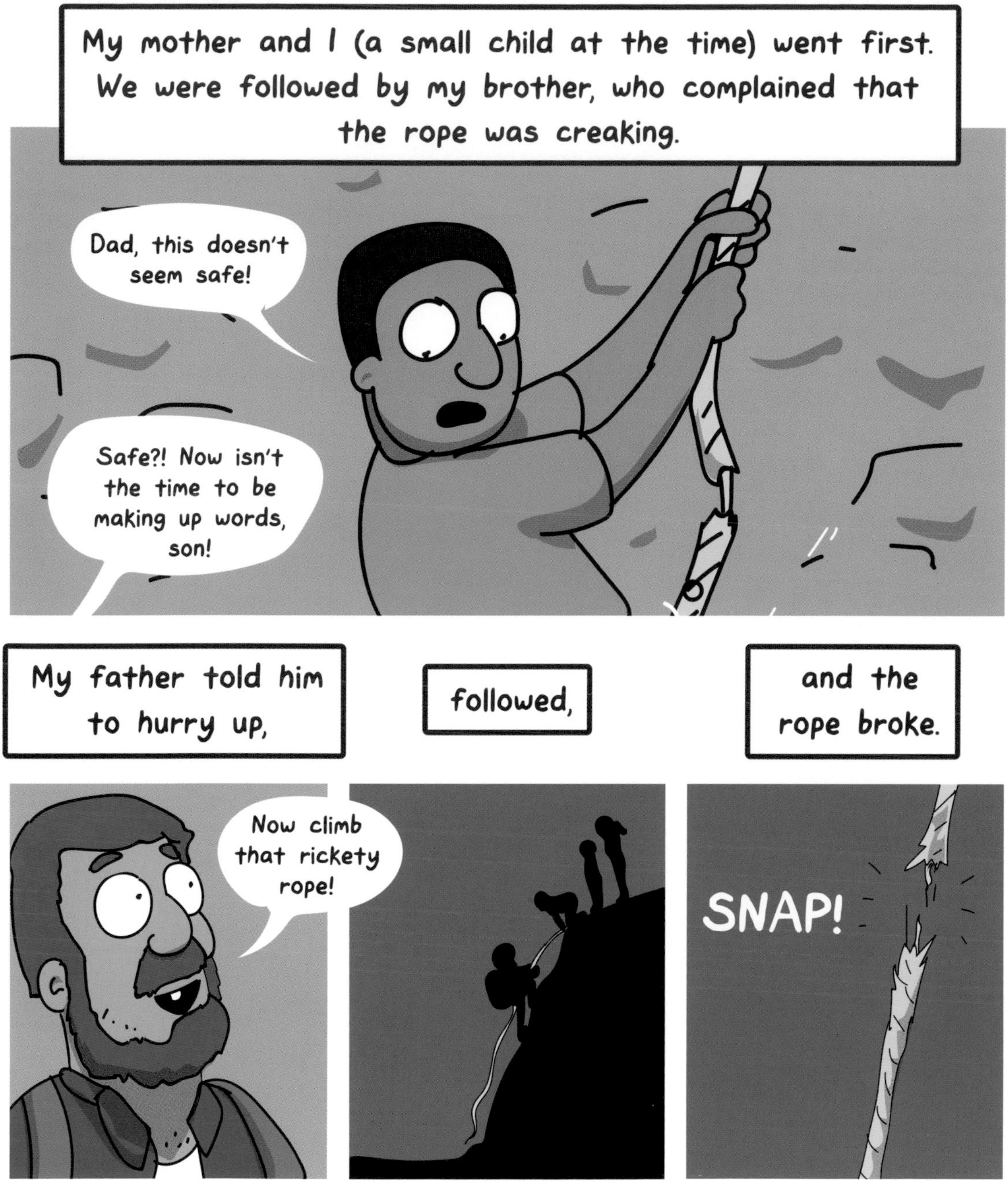
My mother and I (a small child at the time) went first. We were followed by my brother, who complained that the rope was creaking.
Dad, this doesn't seem safe!
Safe?! Now isn't the time to be making up words, son!
My father told him to hurry up,
Now climb that rickety rope!
followed,
and the rope broke.
SNAP!

Apparently, his last word, as he hurtled through the air, was

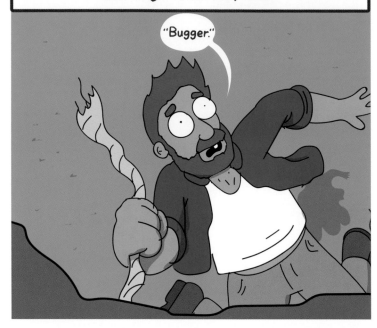

This being St. Helena, all the normal doctors had gone to bed by that time. However, a prolonged search in the empty hospital turned up two young men who claimed to be able to operate an X-ray machine.

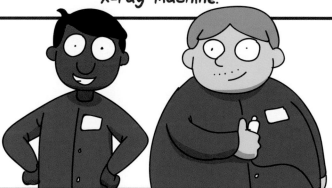

We never asked who they were, but in following years have come to the general conclusion that they must have been employed to sweep the floor.

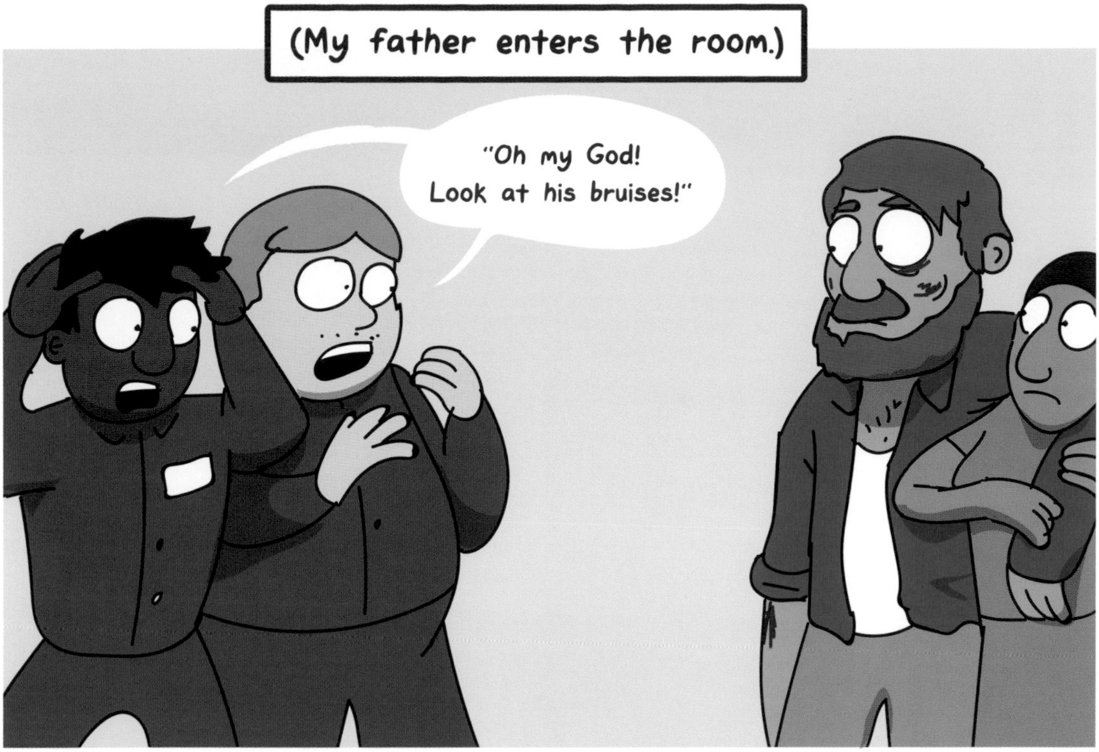
(My father enters the room.)
"Oh my God! Look at his bruises!"

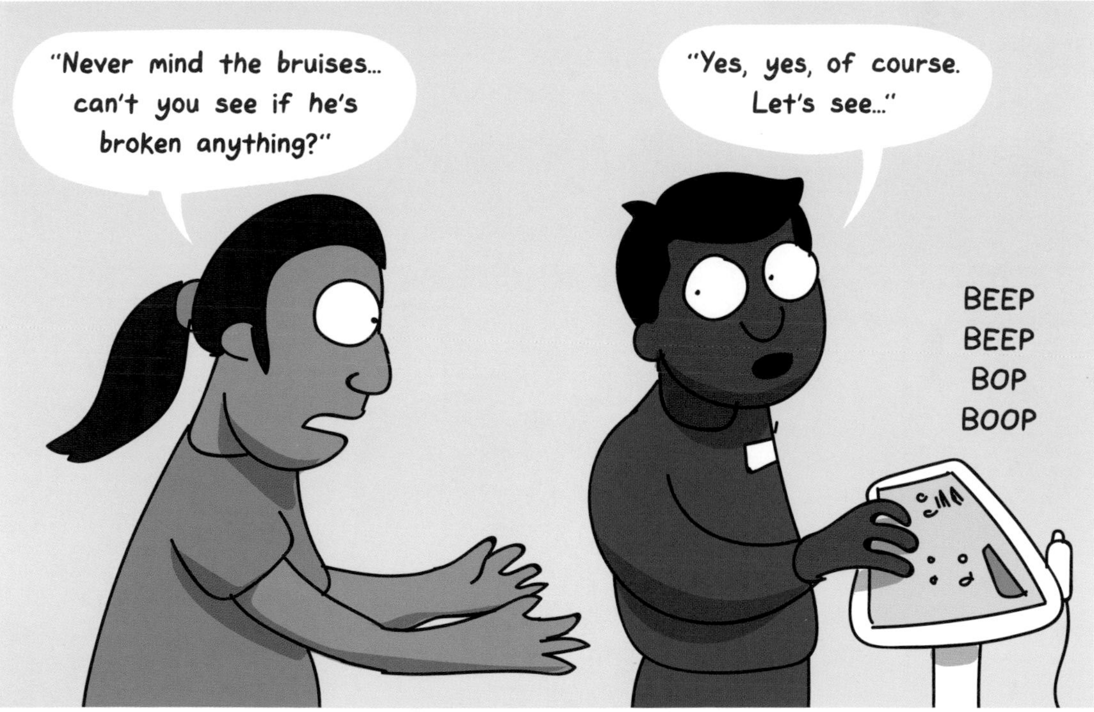
"Never mind the bruises... can't you see if he's broken anything?"
"Yes, yes, of course. Let's see..."
BEEP
BEEP
BOP
BOOP

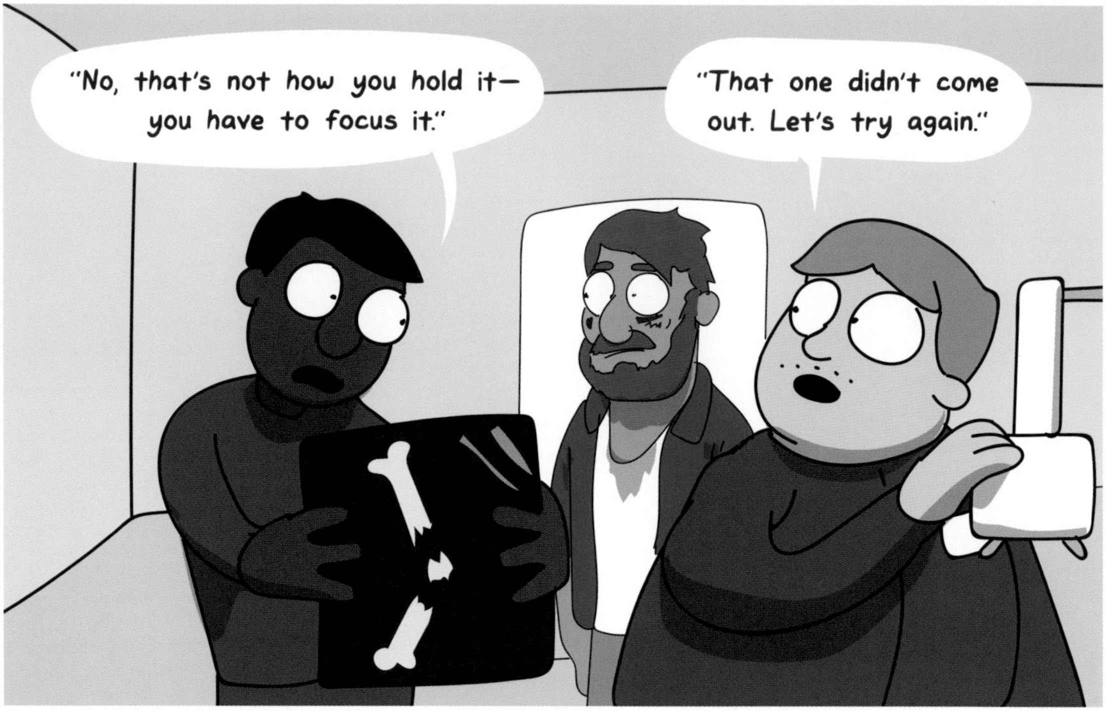
"No, that's not how you hold it—you have to focus it."
"That one didn't come out. Let's try again."

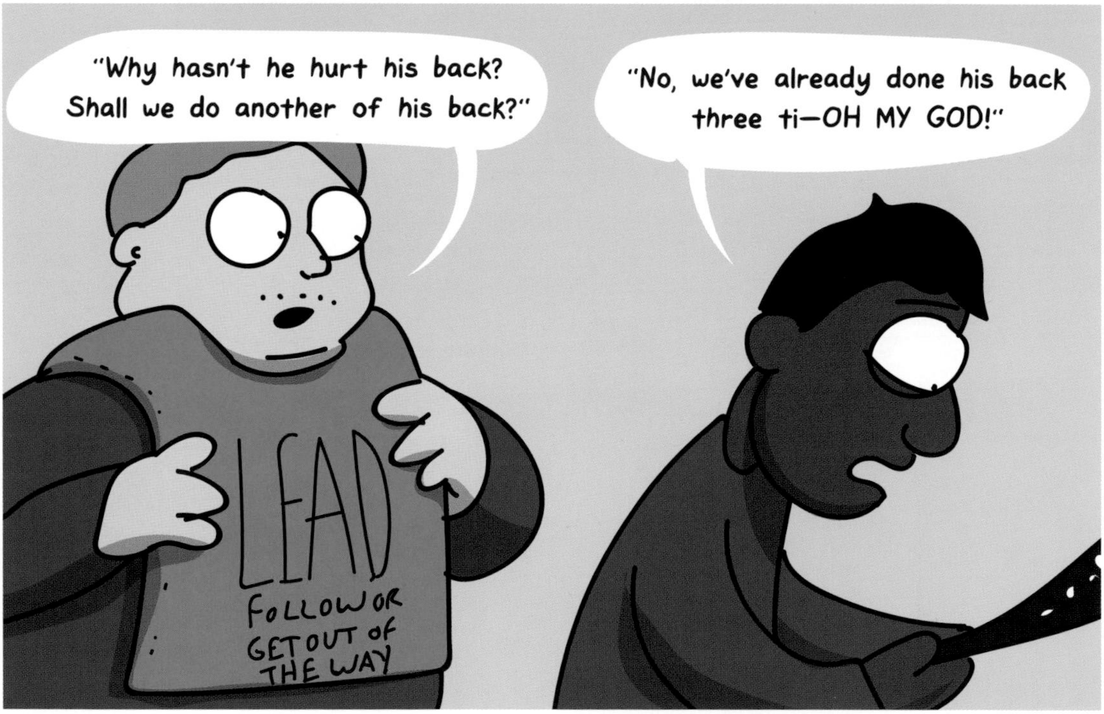
"Why hasn't he hurt his back? Shall we do another of his back?"
"No, we've already done his back three ti—OH MY GOD!"
LEAD
FOLLOW OR
GET OUT OF
THE WAY

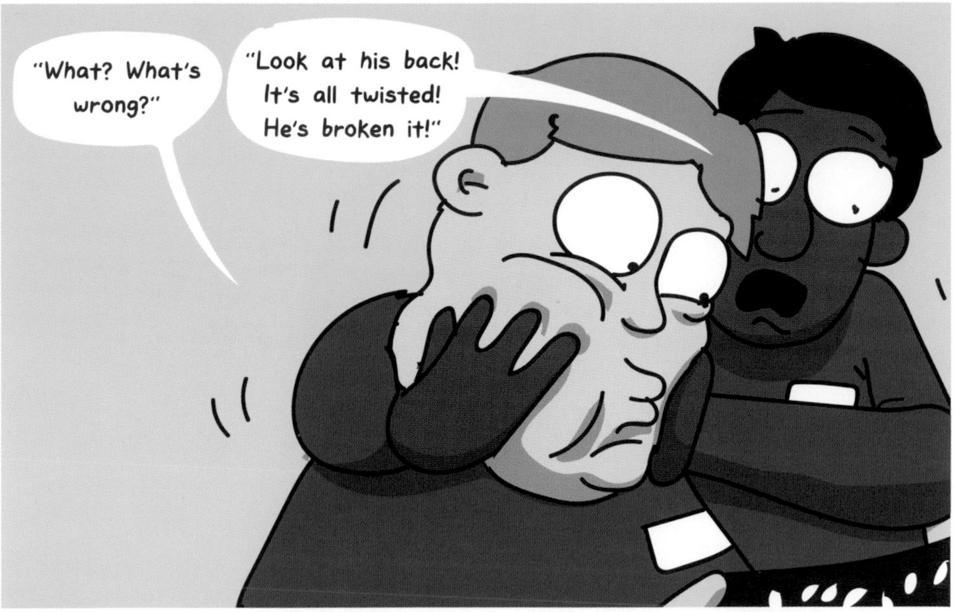
"What? What's wrong?"
"Look at his back! It's all twisted! He's broken it!"

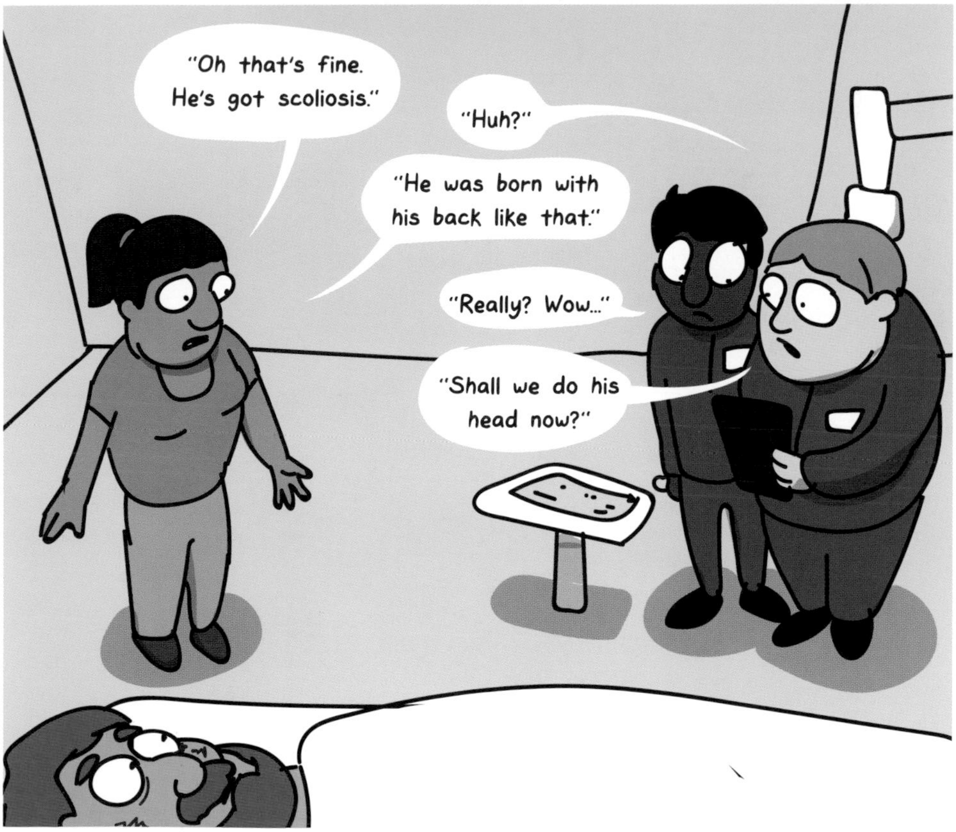
"Oh that's fine. He's got scoliosis."
"Huh?"
"He was born with his back like that."
"Really? Wow..."
"Shall we do his head now?"

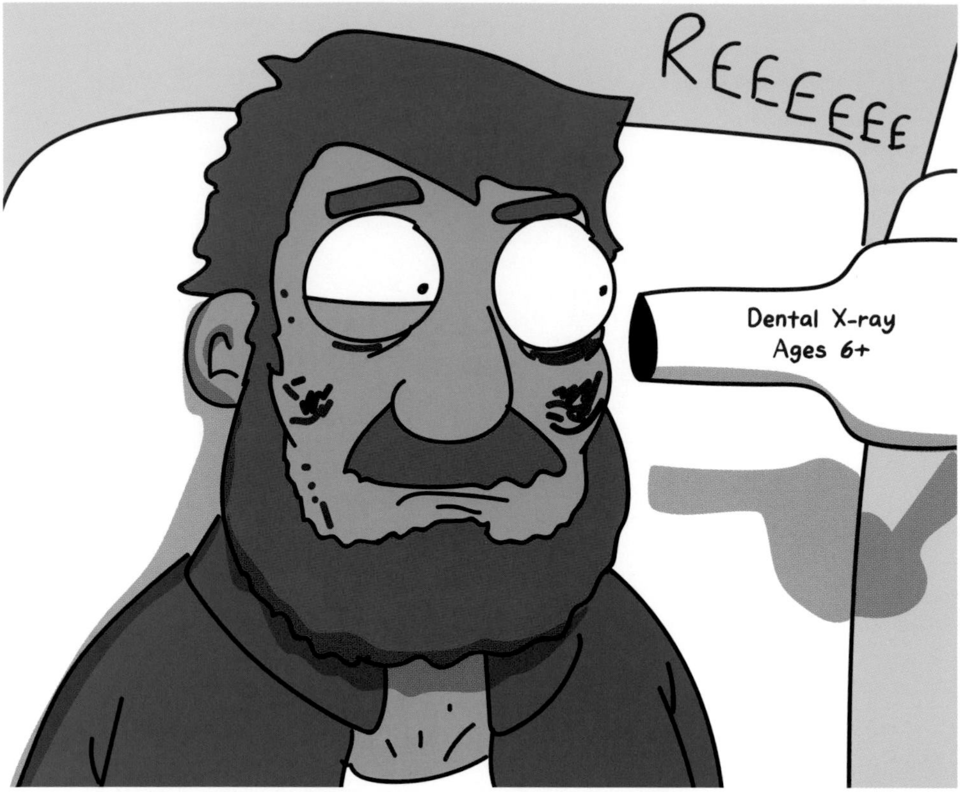
REEEEEEE
Dental X-ray
Ages 6+

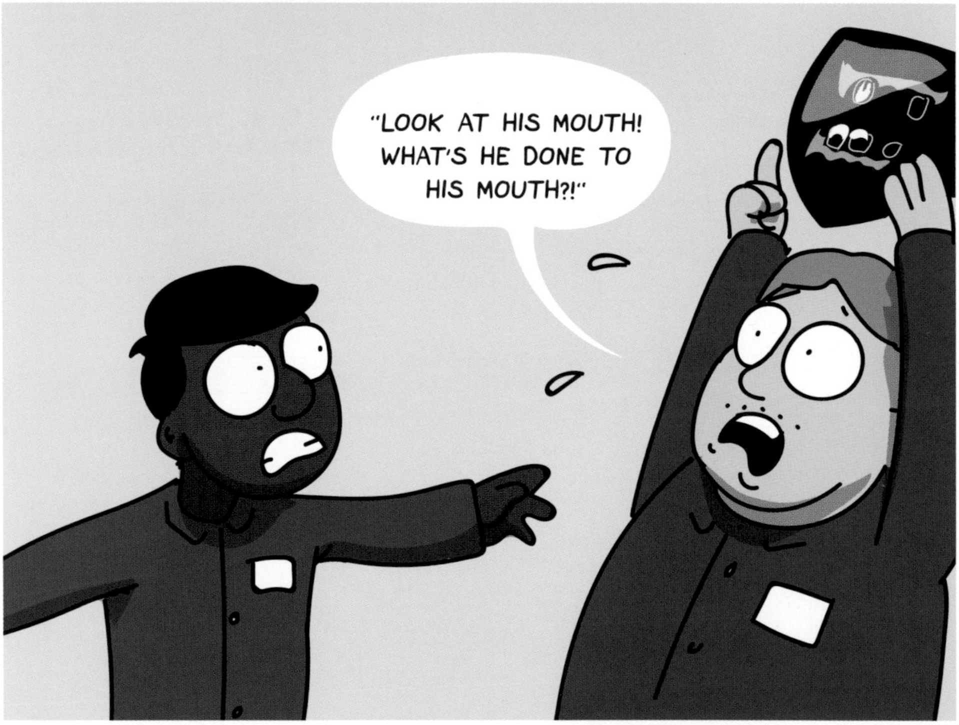
"LOOK AT HIS MOUTH! WHAT'S HE DONE TO HIS MOUTH?!"

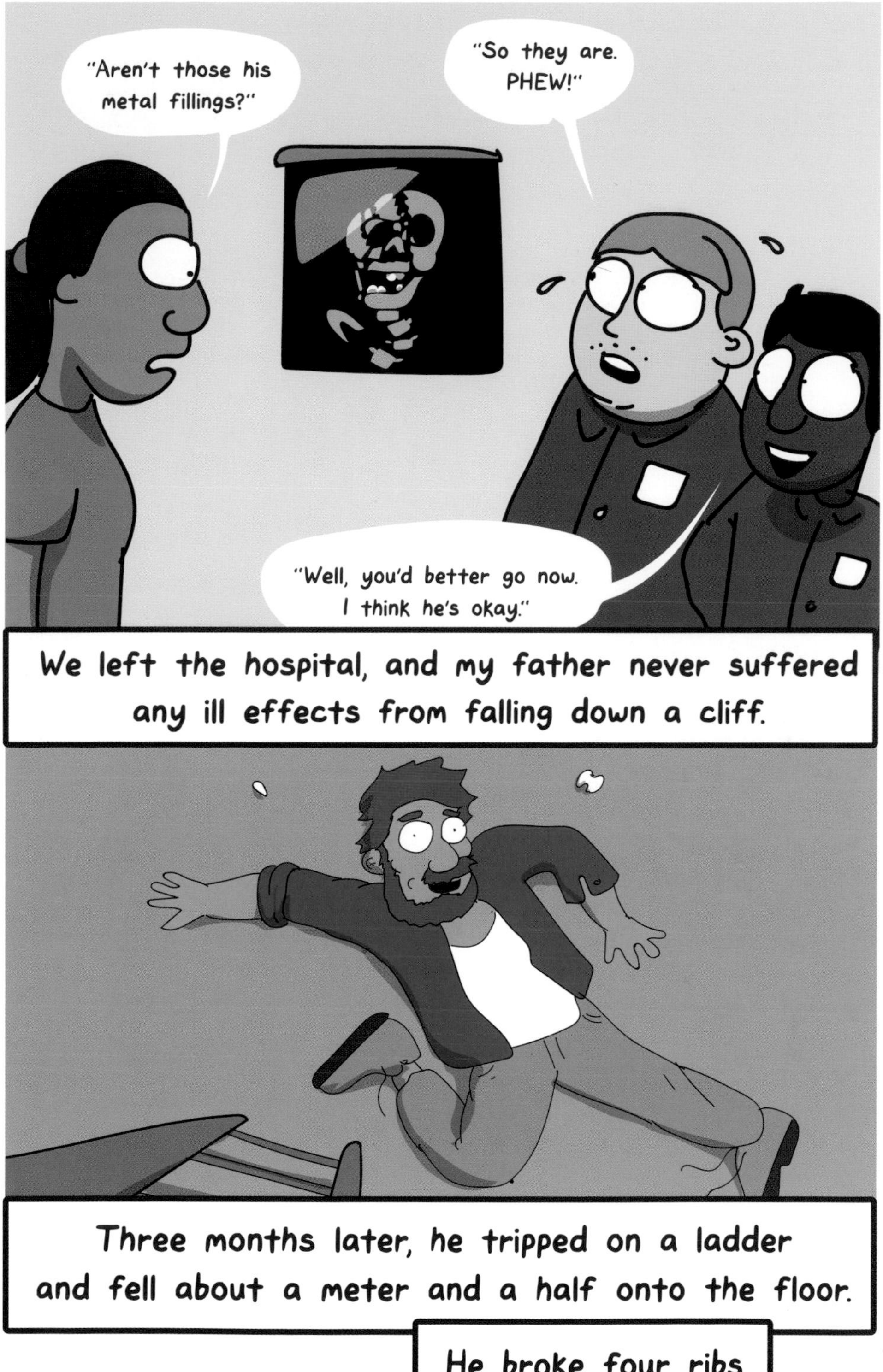
"Aren't those his metal fillings?"
"So they are. PHEW!"
"Well, you'd better go now. I think he's okay."
We left the hospital, and my father never suffered any ill effects from falling down a cliff.
Three months later, he tripped on a ladder and fell about a meter and a half onto the floor.
He broke four ribs.

CHAPTER 24

# THE SHARK THAT WENT NUTS

told by Katie

One day at the beach, I was with my friends and we were all hanging out in the shallows near a cliff by the shore.

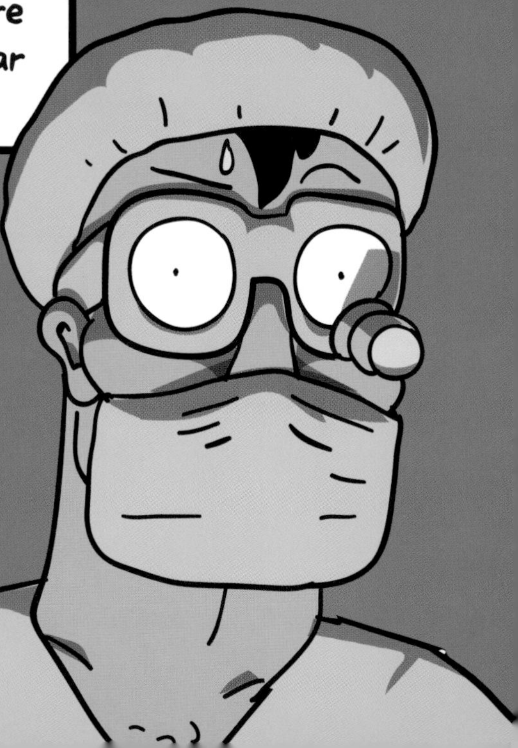

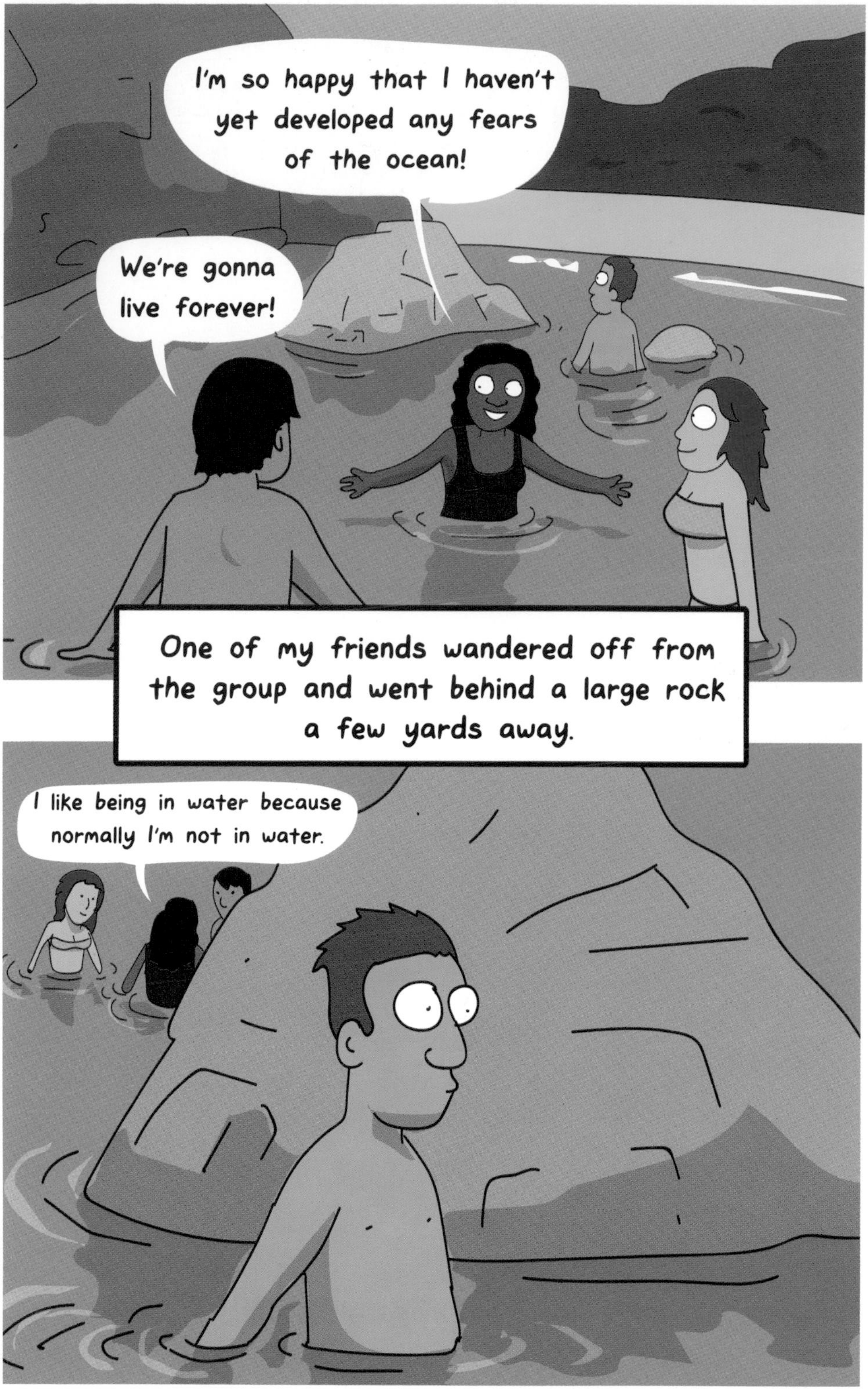
I'm so happy that I haven't yet developed any fears of the ocean!
We're gonna live forever!
One of my friends wandered off from the group and went behind a large rock a few yards away.
I like being in water because normally I'm not in water.

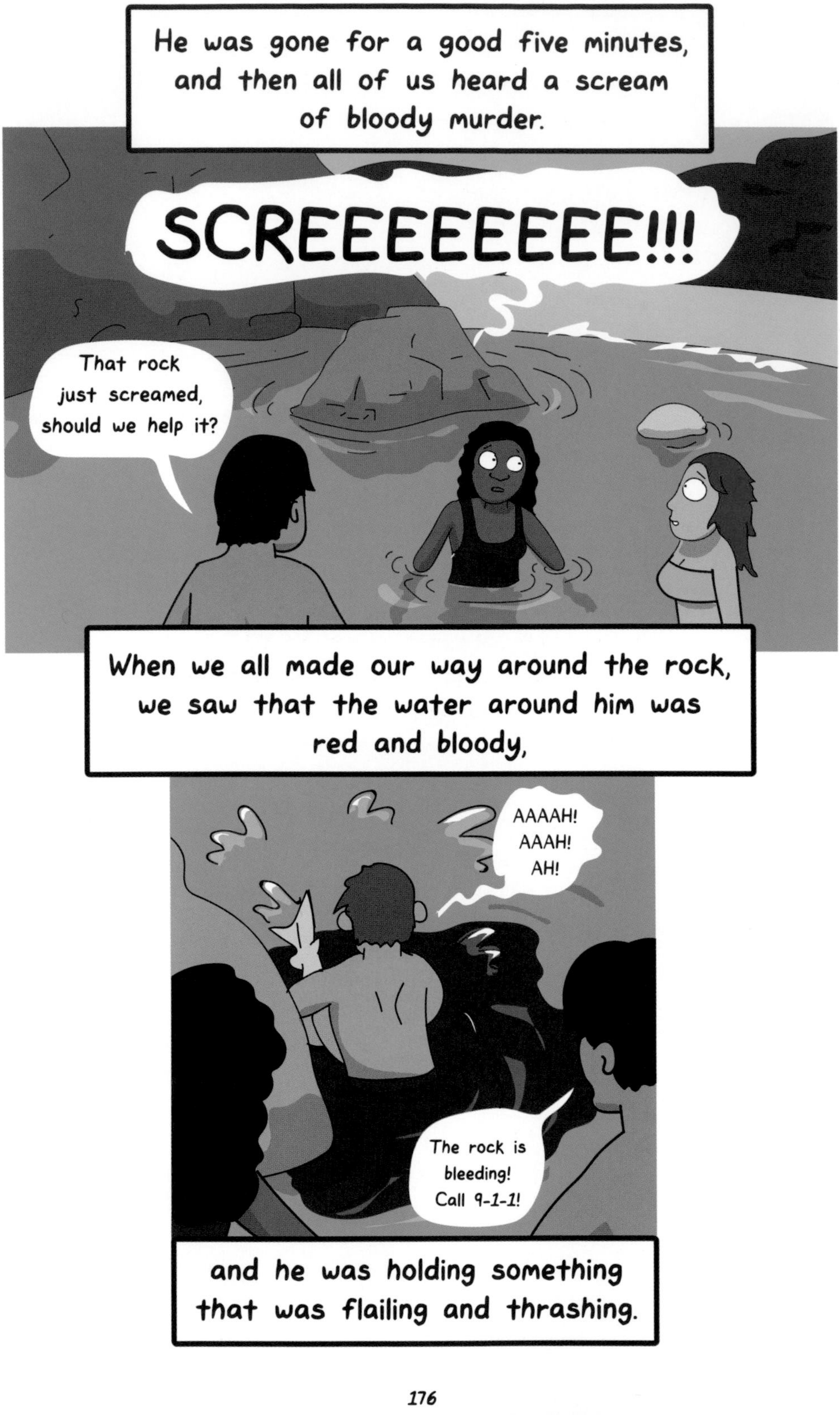
He was gone for a good five minutes, and then all of us heard a scream of bloody murder.
SCREEEEEEEEE!!!
That rock just screamed, should we help it?
When we all made our way around the rock, we saw that the water around him was red and bloody,
AAAAH! AAAH! AH!
The rock is bleeding! Call 9-1-1!
and he was holding something that was flailing and thrashing.

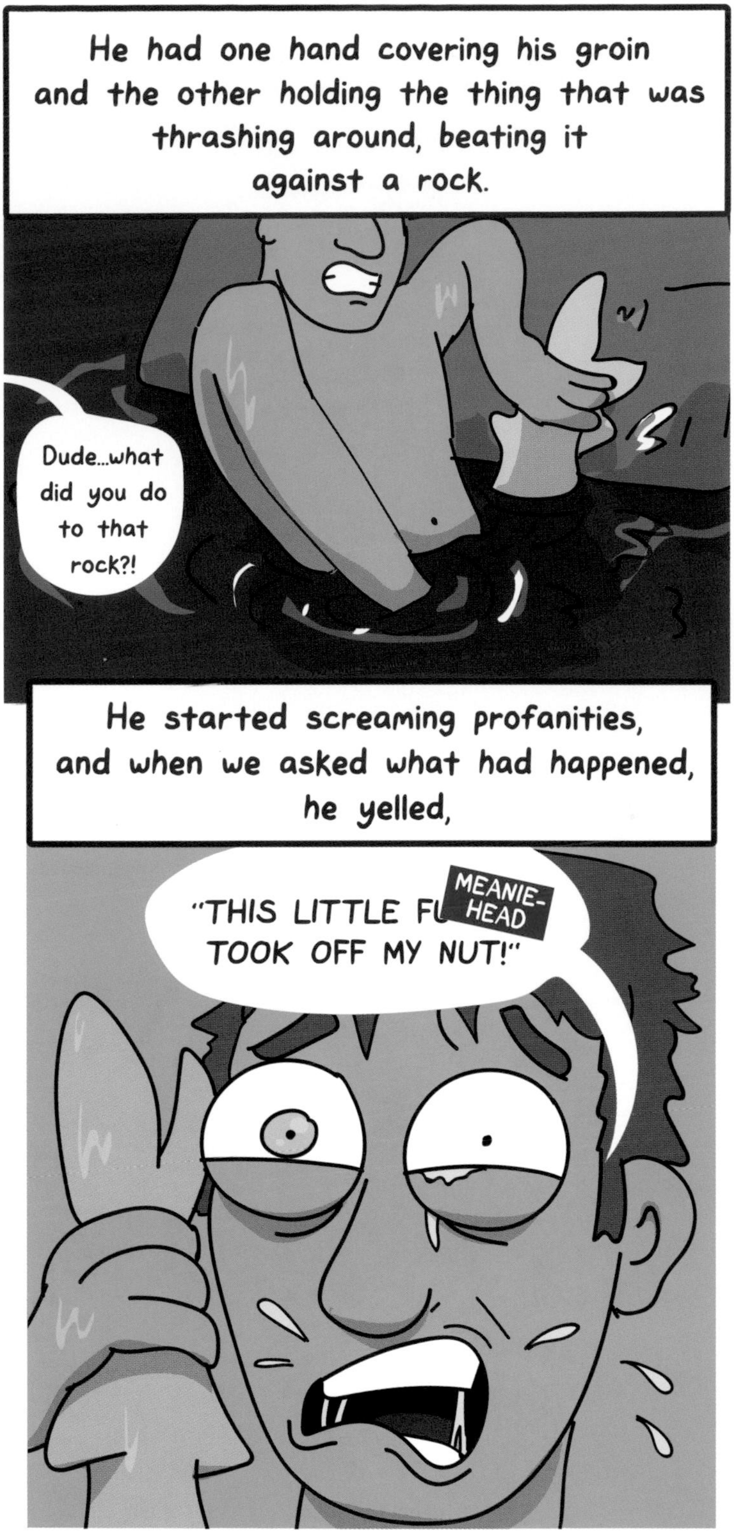
He had one hand covering his groin and the other holding the thing that was thrashing around, beating it against a rock.
Dude...what did you do to that rock?!
He started screaming profanities, and when we asked what had happened, he yelled,
"THIS LITTLE FU MEANIE-HEAD TOOK OFF MY NUT!"

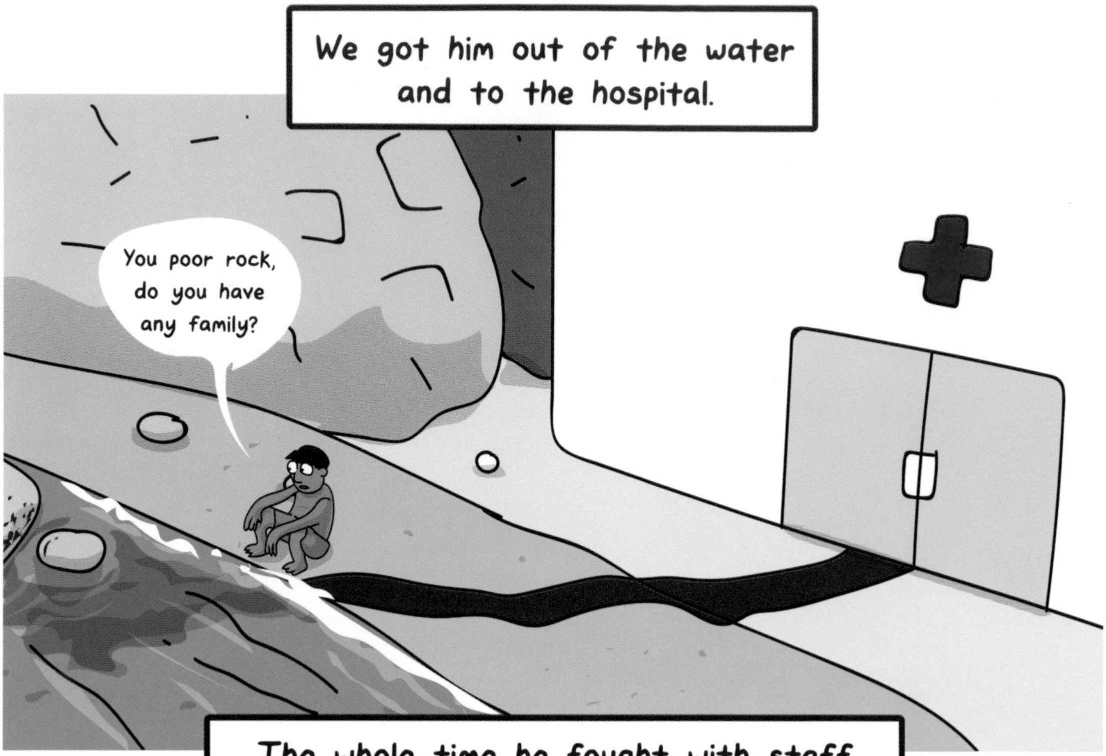
We got him out of the water and to the hospital.
You poor rock, do you have any family?

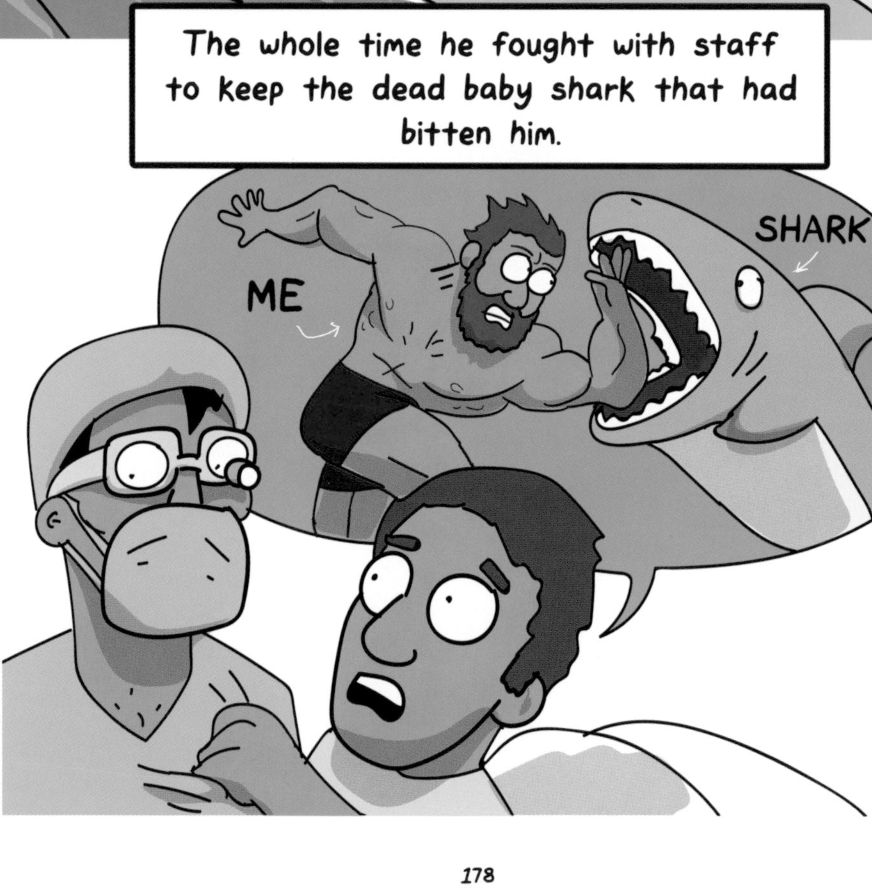
The whole time he fought with staff to keep the dead baby shark that had bitten him.
ME
SHARK

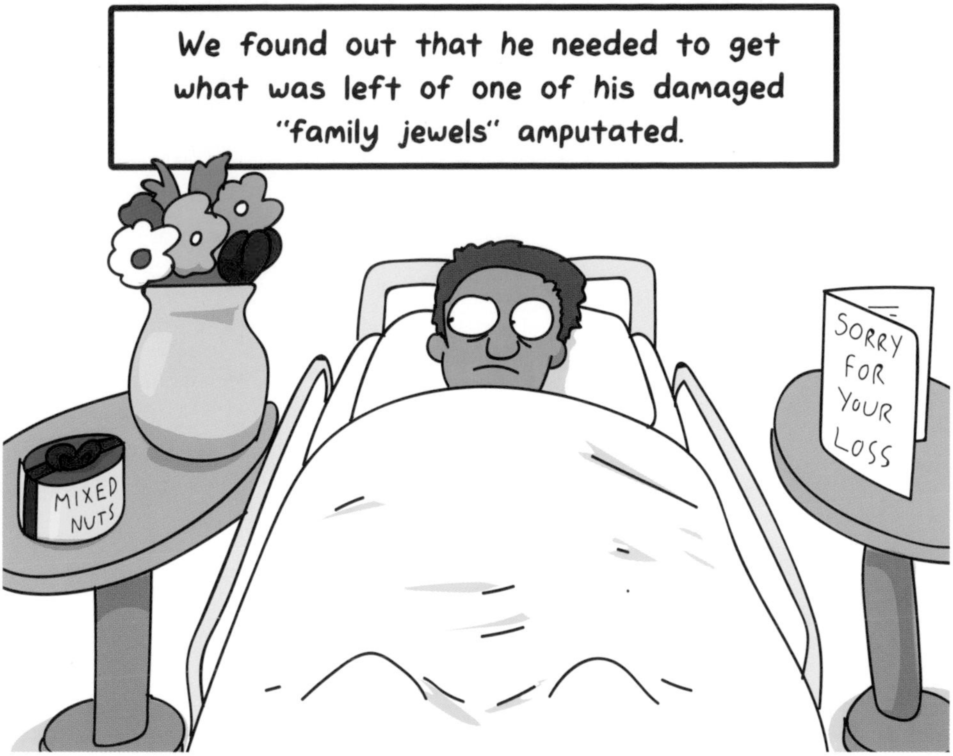
We found out that he needed to get what was left of one of his damaged "family jewels" amputated.
MIXED NUTS
SORRY FOR YOUR LOSS

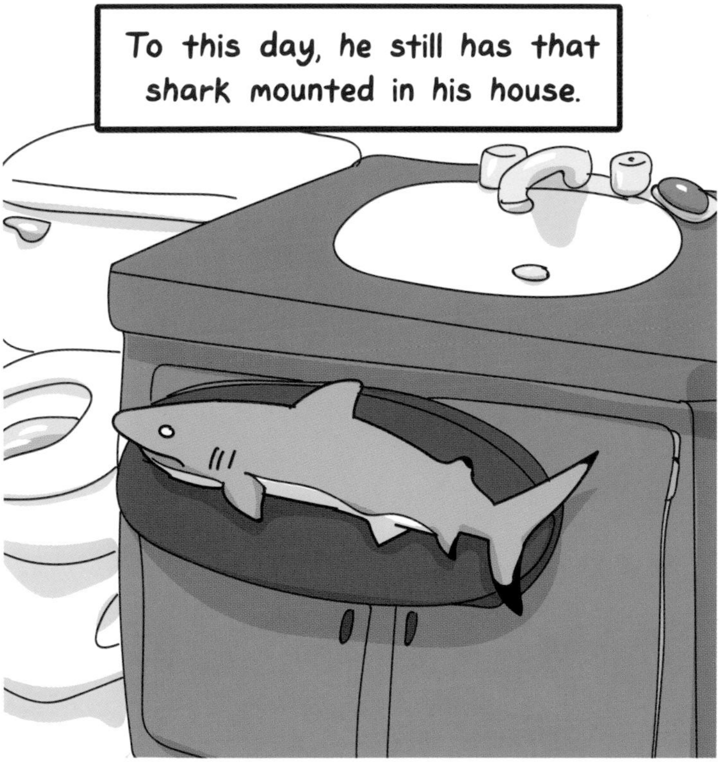
To this day, he still has that shark mounted in his house.

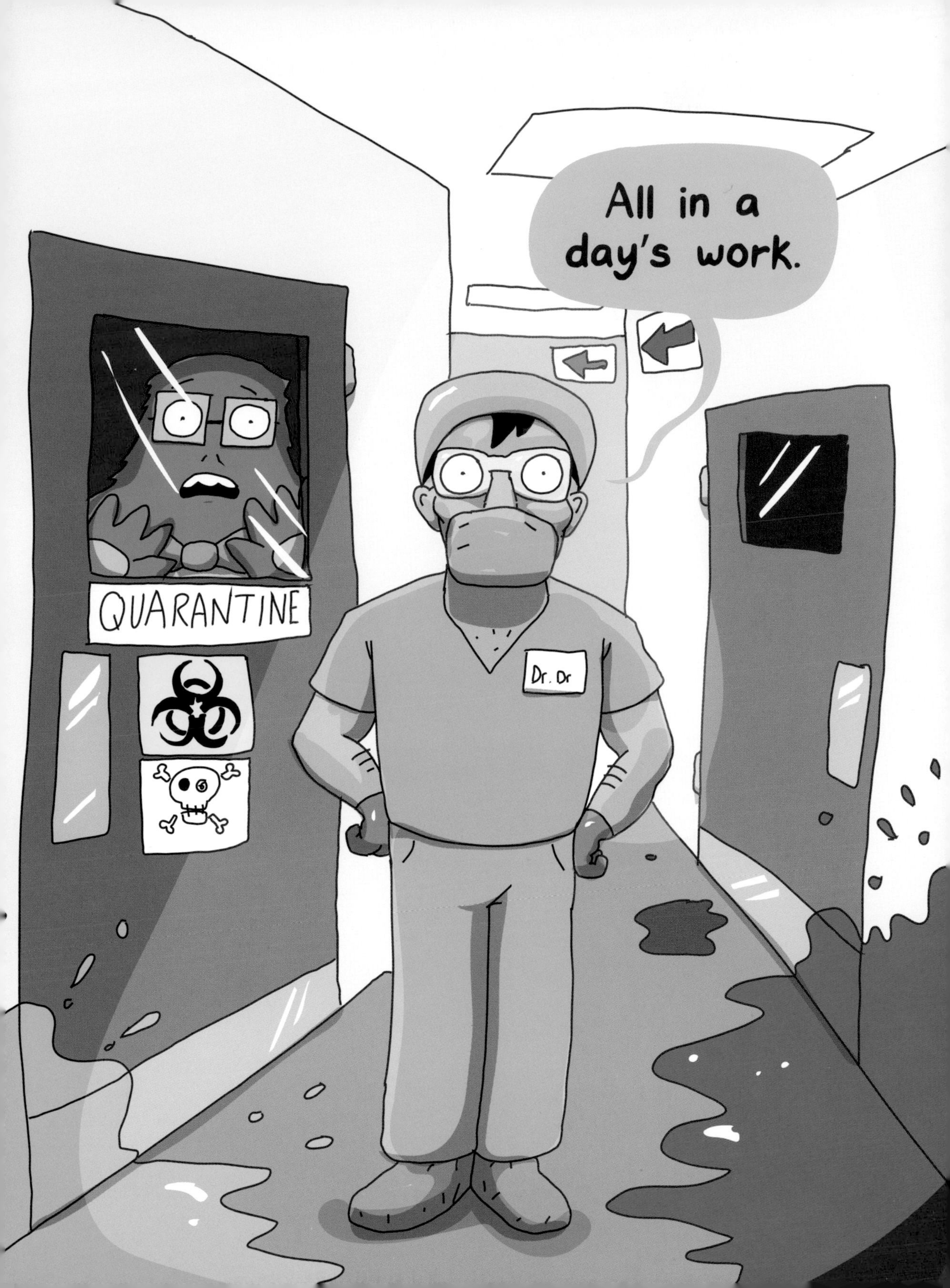
All in a day's work.
QUARANTINE
Dr. Dr

**How I Broke Up with My Colon**



Andrews McMeel Publishing
a division of Andrews McMeel Universal
1130 Walnut Street, Kansas City, Missouri 64106

www.andrewsmcmeel.com

20 21 22 23 24 TEN 10 9 8 7 6 5 4 3 2 1
ISBN: 978-1-5248-5405-8
Library of Congress Control Number: 2019943828

Editor: Lucas Wetzel
Art Director/Designer: Diane Marsh
Production Editor: Amy Strassner
Production Manager: Chuck Harper

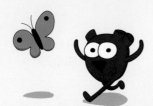